Advanced Synthesis and Medical Applications of Calcium Phosphates

Calcium phosphate materials are used in many medical and dental applications. *Advanced Synthesis and Medical Applications of Calcium Phosphates* covers the structure, chemistry, synthesis, and properties of both natural and synthetic calcium-based biomaterials and details a variety of medical applications.

- Depicts the latest advances in using calcium phosphates in bone regeneration and tissue engineering
- Includes the latest generation of regenerative biomaterials with an integrated perspective combining both research and clinical issues
- Provides an understanding of the clinical targets and requirements for regenerative medicine

Detailing fundamentals through applications, this book helps biomaterials researchers to better understand the clinical targets and requirements for use of these materials for optimal synthesis and development.

Emerging Materials and Technologies

Series Editor: Boris I. Kharissov

The *Emerging Materials and Technologies* series is devoted to highlighting publications centered on emerging advanced materials and novel technologies. Attention is paid to those newly discovered or applied materials with potential to solve pressing societal problems and improve quality of life, corresponding to environmental protection, medicine, communications, energy, transportation, advanced manufacturing, and related areas.

The series takes into account that, under present strong demands for energy, material, and cost savings, as well as heavy contamination problems and worldwide pandemic conditions, the area of emerging materials and related scalable technologies is a highly interdisciplinary field, with the need for researchers, professionals, and academics across the spectrum of engineering and technological disciplines. The main objective of this book series is to attract more attention to these materials and technologies and invite conversation among the international R&D community.

Chemistry of Dehydrogenation Reactions and Its Applications
Edited by Syed Shahabuddin, Rama Gaur, and Nandini Mukherjee

Biosorbents: Diversity, Bioprocessing, and Applications
Edited by Pramod Kumar Mahish, Dakeshwar Kumar Verma, and Shailesh Kumar Jadhav

Principles and Applications of Nanotherapeutics
Imalka Munaweera and Piumika Yapa

Energy Materials: A Circular Economy Approach
Edited by Surinder Singh, Suresh Sundaramuthy, Alex Ibhadon, Faisal Khan, Sushil Kansal, and S.K. Mehta

Tribological Aspects of Additive Manufacturing
Edited by Rashi Tyagi, Ranvijay Kumar, and Nishant Ranjan

Emerging Materials and Technologies for Bone Repair and Regeneration
Edited by Ashok Kumar, Sneha Singh, and Prerna Singh

Mechanics of Auxetic Materials and Structures
Farzad Ebrahimi

Nanomaterials for Sustainable Hydrogen Production and Storage
Edited by Jude A. Okolie, Emmanuel I. Epelle, Alivia Mukherjee, and Alaa El Din Mahmoud

Calcium-Based Materials: Processing, Characterization, and Applications
Edited by S.S. Nanda, Jitendra Pal Singh, Sanjeev Gautam, and Dong Kee Yi

Advanced Synthesis and Medical Applications of Calcium Phosphates
Edited by S.S. Nanda, Jitendra Pal Singh, Sanjeev Gautam, and Dong Kee Yi

For more information about this series, please visit:
www.routledge.com/Emerging-Materials-and-Technologies/book-series/CRCEMT

Advanced Synthesis and Medical Applications of Calcium Phosphates

Edited by
S.S. Nanda
Jitendra Pal Singh
Sanjeev Gautam
Dong Kee Yi

CRC Press
Taylor & Francis Group
Boca Raton London New York

CRC Press is an imprint of the
Taylor & Francis Group, an **informa** business

Designed cover image: © Sanjeev Gautam

First edition published 2024
by CRC Press
2385 NW Executive Center Drive, Suite 320, Boca Raton FL 33431

and by CRC Press
4 Park Square, Milton Park, Abingdon, Oxon, OX14 4RN

CRC Press is an imprint of Taylor & Francis Group, LLC

Library of Congress Cataloging-in-Publication Data

Names: Nanda, S. S. (Sitansu Sekhar), editor. | Singh, Jitendra Pal, editor. | Gautam, Sanjeev, editor. | Yi, Dong Kee, editor.
Title: Advanced synthesis and medical applications of calcium phosphates / edited by S.S. Nanda, Jitendra Pal Singh, Sanjeev Gautam, and Dong Kee Yi.
Other titles: Emerging materials and technologies.
Description: First edition. | Boca Raton, FL : CRC Press, 2024. | Series: Emerging materials and technologies | Includes bibliographical references and index.
Identifiers: LCCN 2023052093 (print) | LCCN 2023052094 (ebook) | ISBN 9781032419633 (hardback) | ISBN 9781032419657 (paperback) | ISBN 9781003360605 (ebook)
Subjects: MESH: Calcium Phosphates--therapeutic use | Biocompatible Materials--therapeutic use | Tissue Engineering--methods | Regenerative Medicine--methods
Classification: LCC R857.T55 (print) | LCC R857.T55 (ebook) | NLM QT 37 | DDC 610.28--dc23/eng/20240207
LC record available at https://lccn.loc.gov/2023052093
LC ebook record available at https://lccn.loc.gov/2023052094

ISBN: 978-1-032-41963-3 (hbk)
ISBN: 978-1-032-41965-7 (pbk)
ISBN: 978-1-003-36060-5 (ebk)

DOI: 10.1201/9781003360605

Typeset in Nimbus Roman
by KnowledgeWorks Global Ltd.

Dedication

In homage to the curious minds of young researchers,
Whose unyielding passion ignites the torch of discovery.

To the preservation and nurturing of our environment,
A commitment to safeguarding the home we share.

And to the realm of smart materials innovation,
A beacon guiding humanity towards a brighter, sustainable future.

Contents

Preface

This volume delves into the realm of calcium phosphates and their extensive applications within the realm of medicine. The fundamental focus of this book revolves around introducing calcium phosphates and elucidating their significance in medical contexts. The pages ahead unfold a thorough exploration of various facets, all tailored towards realizing the core objectives of this book.

Within these chapters, we embark on an enlightening journey through the forefront of knowledge, encapsulating the latest strides in the utilization of calcium phosphates for the advancement of bone regeneration and tissue engineering. By intertwining research intricacies with clinical dimensions, this book strives to present a holistic perspective on the cutting-edge generation of regenerative biomaterials.

One of the foremost objectives of this endeavor is to bridge the gap between research and practice. By addressing both the innovative developments in this field and their direct implications for clinical settings, this volume aspires to foster a deeper comprehension among biomaterials researchers. In essence, it aids researchers in aligning their pursuits with the tangible needs and aspirations of regenerative medicine.

As we embark on this literary expedition, the chapters within not only serve to expand our knowledge base but also encourage us to envision a future where calcium phosphates play an increasingly pivotal role in shaping the landscape of medical solutions. This book is more than a compilation of information; it is a dynamic resource designed to inspire new perspectives and cultivate a synergistic relationship between scientific innovation and healthcare outcomes.

May the following pages kindle curiosity, ignite inspiration, and serve as a beacon guiding us towards the realization of novel possibilities in the fascinating realm of calcium phosphates and their diverse medical applications.

Editors

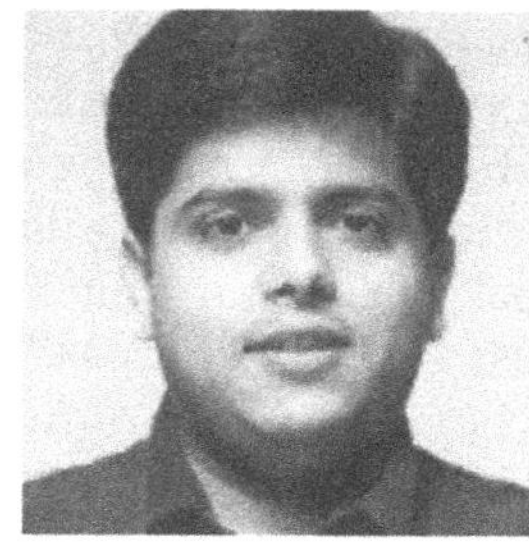

S.S. Nanda, PhD, was born in Odisha, India, and earned a BPharm (2007) and MPharm (2009) in pharmacy at Biju Patnaik University of Technology, Odisha. In 2009, he became an Assistant Professor at Vikas College of Pharmaceutical Sciences, Suryapet, Telengana. In 2012, he moved to Gachon University and earned a PhD (2015) in bionanotechnology, working with Prof. Dong Kee Yi. He has authored and co-authored more than 50 peer-reviewed international journal articles and worked as an inventor for one patent. In 2015, he became an Assistant Professor at Myongji University. His research interests include tissue engineering and applications of materials in nanomedicine.

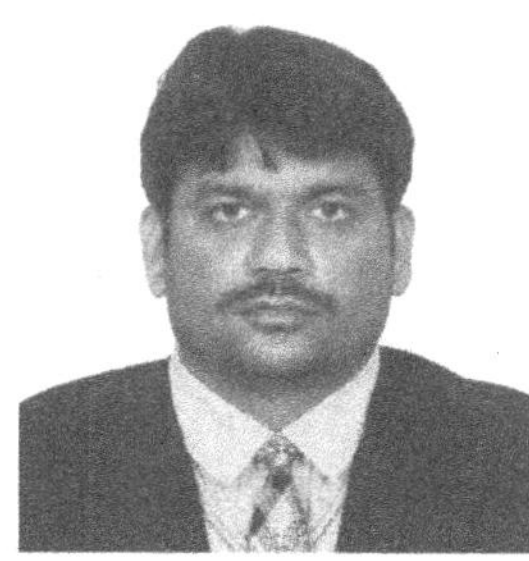

Jitendra Pal Singh, PhD, is a Ramanujan Fellow in the Department of Sciences (Physics), Manav Rachna University, Faridabad, Haryana, India. In 2010, he earned a PhD at Govind Ballabh Pant University of Agriculture and Technology, Pantnagar, Uttarakhand. He has worked at Pohang Accelerator Laboratory, Pohang, Republic of Korea, and the Korea Institute of Science and Technology, Seoul, Korea (2014–2022); Inter-University Accelerator Centre, New Delhi (2010–2011); Taiwan SPIN Research Centre, National Chung Cheng University, Taiwan (2011–2012); and Krishna Engineering College, Ghaziabad, India (2012–2014). His research interests are irradiation studies in nanoferrites, thin films, and magnetic multilayers. In May 2022, he joined the faculty of the Department of Sciences (Physics), Manav Rachna University, Faridabad, India. He is actively working on the synthesis of ferrite nanoparticles and thin films and determining the magnetic, optical, and dielectric responses of ferrites. He also studies the irradiation and implantation effects of ferrite thin films and nanoparticles. Dr. Singh has authored one book, *Ion Beam Induced Defects and Their Effects in Oxide Materials* (Springer, 2022), and edited five books: *Ferrite Nanostructured Magnetic Materials* (Elsevier, 2023); *Application of Ferrite Nanostructures* (Elsevier, 2023); *Oxide for Magnetic Applications* (Elsevier, 2023); *Defect Induced Magnetism in Oxide Semiconductors* (Elsevier, 2023); and *Sol-Gel Method: Recent Advances* (In Tech, 2023). He is a Guest Editor for several journals, including *Journal of Alloys and Compounds* and *RSC Advances*. He is also a Topic Editor for the journal *Magnetism* (*MDPI*) and the Founding Editor-in-Chief of the journal *Prabha Materials Science Letters*. He has authored and co-authored more than 150 peer-reviewed international journal articles related to ferrites, carbonates, X-ray absorption spectroscopy, and X-ray imaging.

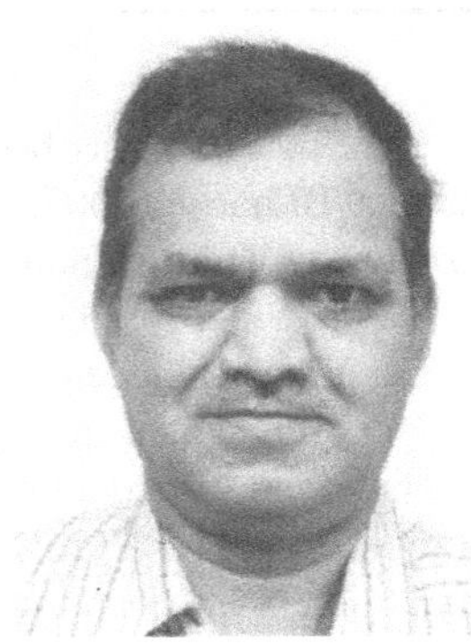

Sanjeev Gautam, PhD, leads an independent research group, the Advanced Functional Materials Laboratory, at Dr. S.S. Bhatnagar University Institute of Chemical Engineering and Technology, Panjab University, Chandigarh, India. He has more than 25 years' experience with more than 161 international publications (h-index = 31 with 4000+ citations). He earned a PhD (2007) in condensed matter physics at the Centre of Advanced Study in Physics, Panjab University. He worked as a grid computing administrator in the CMS (LHC, Geneva) research project (MCSE, 2001–2007). As a beamline scientist at the Korea Institute of Science and Technology, South Korea (2007–2014), he was awarded a star post-doc. At Panjab University, as an Assistant Professor (2014–present), he has received international and national grants in nanotechnology, sustainable energy, food technology, catalysts, environmental safety, and administrative duties. Dr. Gautam has supervised seven PhD students and 32+ master's theses and promoted undergraduate research at Panjab University. He serves as an editorial board member for *Scientific Reports* (Nature Publications), *Materials Letters* and *Materials Letters: X* (Elsevier), and *Heliyon* (Cell).

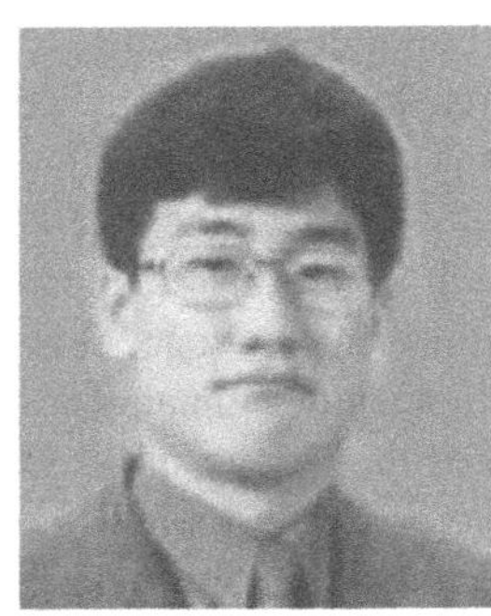

Dong Kee Yi, PhD, earned a PhD in materials science and engineering in 2003 at the Gwangju Institute of Science and Technology (Korea). He went through his post-doc fellow seasons at Brown University and IBN at Singapore from 2003 to 2005. He worked as a Senior Scientist at the Samsung Advanced Institute of Technology from 2005 to 2007. From 2007 to 2013 he was on the faculty of the Department of Bionanotechnology, Gachon University (Korea). In 2013, he joined the faculty of the Department of Chemistry, Myongji University. He has edited one book, *Nanobiomaterials: Development and Applications* (CRC Press, Taylor & Francis, 2013). He has authored or co-authored more than 150 peer-reviewed international journal articles and worked as an inventor for 33 international patents. He serves on the editorial board for *ISRN Nanotechnology* and is a reviewer for the journals of leading scientific societies, including the American Chemical Society, the Royal Society of Chemistry, and the American Institute of Physics. He also works as a research/technology evaluator and on several advisory panels for the Chinese, Korean, and Romanian governments. He also is a consultant for industrial organizations in Korea.

1 Biocompatibility of Natural Materials (Calcium Phosphates)

Sanjeev Gautam and Lidiya Sonowal
Advanced Functional Materials Laboratory, Dr. S.S. Bhatnagar University Institute of Chemical Engineering and Technology, Panjab University, Chandigarh, India

1.1 INTRODUCTION

Biomaterials, are compounds found in remedial or diagnostic systems that are brought into correspondence with tissue or bodily fluids but are not meals or medications [1]. They are employed in a variety of medicinal arrangements such as transdermal patches for the skin and covering for pills and pellets [2]. Originally, implanted devices that are intended to reside inside a person for a lengthy period have been subject to biocompatibility testing. Therefore, a compilation of negative qualities was employed to define biocompatibility when choosing elements or on occasions when developing new ones. These qualities included non-toxicity, non-immunogenicity, non-thrombogenicity, non-carcinogenicity, etc. [3]. With utilization featuring tissue engineering, intrusive detectors, drug administration, and gene transmission systems, therapeutically focused nanotechnological advancement in addition to the relevant devices for medical implants, the implementation of biomaterials has become more varied and intricate, resulting in ambiguity over the processes and requirements for biocompatibility is turning into a major obstacle to the advancement of these new technologies [4].

The emergence of calcium phosphate-based (CaP) biomaterials is bolstered due to their resemblance to bone in terms of constitution. For instance, a CaP in the form of carbonate apatite along with its characteristics, such as being biodegradable, biological activity and osteoconductivity [5]. Through the application of porogens during the manufacturing process of CaP biomaterials, interlinking porosity, another crucial bone characteristic can be added. Despite having these advantageous qualities, CaP biomaterials exhibit a poor fracture resilience and ought not to be used in load-bearing locations [6]. Orthopaedic and orthodontic implants with CaP coverings merge the metal's stiffness with its biological activity. A number of

DOI: 10.1201/9781003360605-1

different kinds of CaP-based biomaterial, including hydroxyapatite (HAp), brushite, tricalcium phosphate, and whitlockite, have been used in medical diagnostics lately. Because of its exceptional qualities, HAp has been explored the most, particularly in tissue engineering [7]. In addition, significant uses for whitlockite, tricalcium phosphate, and brushite have also been employed, which include coatings for dental implants to the treatment of kidney stones [8].

The osteoinductivity of bone, which enables it to heal and replenish itself, is a crucial attribute. Bone morphogenetic proteins (BMPs) and osteogenic proteins like collagen that are found in the matrix of cells are key factors responsible for inducing osteoinductive properties in bone [9]. Substances made of CaP do not promote bone formation on their own but fortunately, these substances can be given osteoinductive characteristics using one of two approaches: in order to trap and concentrate flowing growth factors or osteoprogenitor cells, or to incorporate it with growth factors (BMPs) or biologically active proteins (collage), the CaPs must be designed with the proper geometry, contours, combination of macro- and microporosity, and concavities. The effectiveness of this framework or carriage is impacted by the microporosity/macroporosity, composition, and quantity of particles in the second scenario [10]. In general, CaP is considered having low toxicity, and it is commonly regarded as safe for use in food and medical applications [11]. However, it is essential to note that excessive exposure to high concentrations may still pose some risks [12,13]. The toxicity assessment of CaP has been discussed in the article with reference to several experimental studies.

1.2 TYPES OF CaP

An essential component of maintaining and defending the functioning of the body is bone, a calcified substance. Defects in the bones brought on by injury, ageing, infection, and tumors have a significant impact on individual health and ability to lead normal lives. Bone defects cannot be self healed and have to be guided by the use of biomaterials for its restoration. CaP-based biomaterials encompass a specific place amid the various biomaterials employed for bone healing due to their similarity to the chemical elements and structural elements of native bone tissue [14]. There are different types of CaP, that are used in different biomedical applications as shown in Figure 1.1. Following section is an attempt to review the utilization of various forms

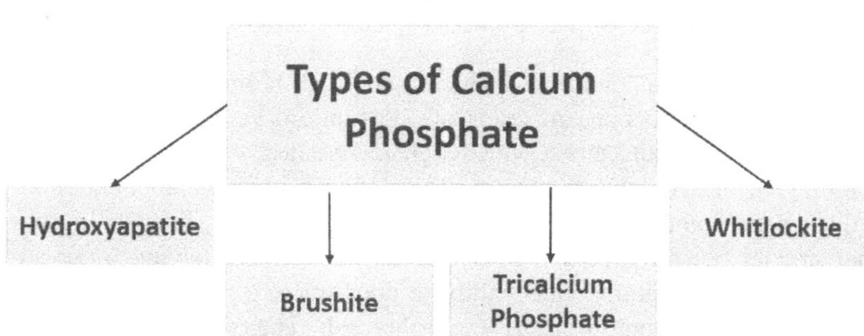

Figure 1.1 Diagram showing different types of calcium phosphate.

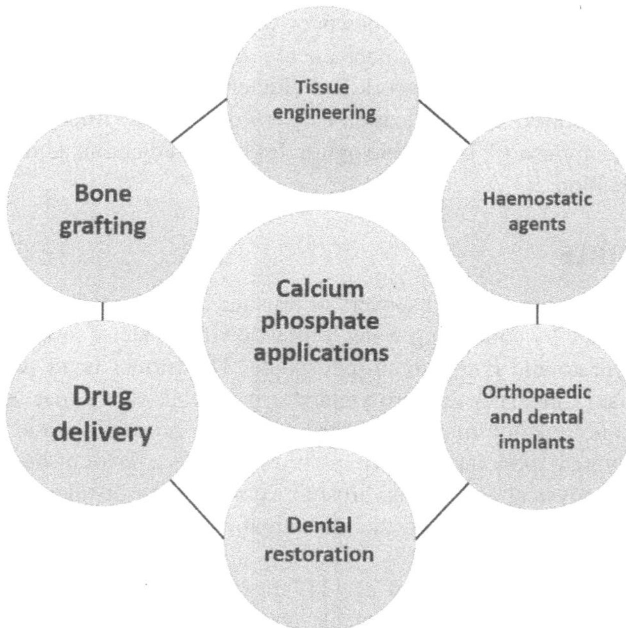

Figure 1.2 Illustration depicting biomedical applications of calcium phosphate.

of CaP in medical uses. Figure 1.2 depicts the various biomedical applications of CaP.

1.2.1 HYDROXYAPATITE

A biomaterial that has received extensive research is hydroxyapatite (HAp), which shares similar chemical properties with the mineral that makes up bones. Additionally, it is bioactive, biocompatible, and stable in physiological fields, making it an appealing substance for a variety of biomedical applications prominently in the orthopaedic fields [15]. HAp can be utilized as frameworks for tissue engineering, coating implants, and the controlled release of medications. Alone, HAp may lack the desired strength and fracture toughness. Doping of the same with various elements may make up for the desired qualities.

By using compressive strength testing and fracture resilience Bhatnagar et al. [16] attempted to study the mechanical strength and demonstrated that by increasing the amount of carbonate, the material's strength during compression and resilience to fracture significantly rises, thus making it a strong candidate for use as a biomaterial in the construction of biomedical implants. Employing 3D gel printing, Shao et al. [17] effectively created permeable HAp scaffolds and demonstrated that the scaffolds have suitable degrading parameters for use in skeletal tissue engineering and have compressive strengths that are better compared to bones with a cancellous structure.

Injectable OAlg-CMCS gel frameworks were created by Ren et al. [18], and demonstrated that they had strong mechanical properties, good injectability, and appropriate dissolution. This framework had efficient antibiotic action toward *E. coli* and *S. aures* when used as a medication delivery device. The findings indicated that a combined gel framework is a viable option for both medication administration and bone tissue creation.

1.2.2 BRUSHITE

Mirtchi and Lematre made the discovery of brushite cements in 1989 [19]. The compounds were made by combining water with a powder made of monocalcium phosphate monohydrate and β-tricalcium phosphate. The former is an acidic CaP, and the later a basic CaP. This mixture yielded a malleable slurry that later hardened in an exothermic reaction to create a hard substance primarily made of dicalcium phosphate dihydrate, popularly known as "brushite". As a result of its capacity to be resorbed under physical conditions, brushite cement has a distinct edge over other CaP cement system like HAp. Further investigations also revealed brushite cement to be biocompatible [20].

In his investigations Zhuang et al. [21] made an effort to restore cranial bone anomalies using innovative biodegradable porous Zn alloy scaffolds with brushite coating and demonstrated that coated Zn alloy had favorable biocompatibility and minimal cytotoxicity. Additionally, it might encourage rabbit BMSCs' osteogenic proliferation and accumulation of calcium in vitro as well as the growth of fresh bones adjacent to the framework in vivo. Furthermore, it was concluded that in order to heal cranial bone defects, the degradable porous Zn alloy framework with brushite coating is indeed promising.

Sudhan et al. [22] synthesized brushite nanoparticles and attempted to determine UA, XN, HXN, and CF simultaneously by electrochemistry using the SWV method. Using the brushite-modified electrode, each of these four purine derivatives was separately determined whilst the presence of other compounds. Considering its low monitoring limits, the manufactured brushite/GCE demonstrated excellent selectivity and sensitivity for both solitary and concurrent voltammetric analysis.

By initiating the polymerization of gelatin while cement setting, a unique dual-setting brushite-gelatin cement was developed by Rodel et al. [23], and demonstrated that the compound exhibited enhanced flexibility and prolonged release of medication.

1.2.3 TRICALCIUM PHOSPHATE

CaP can be easily shaped into complex geometrical shapes and exhibit good biological activity and compatibility. The rate of absorption, however, is minimal. Therefore, tricalcium phosphate (TCP) has been receiving a lot of consideration as an alternative to bone grafts.

Tricalcium phosphate ($Ca_3(PO_4)_2$) demonstrates an atomic ratio of Ca/P of 1.5. It exists in four different forms: the form α is metastable at room temperature and steady between 1120 and 1470 °C; the form α' is steady on and above 1470 °C; the form β is steady on and below 1120 °C; and the form γ is produced under high pressure. During bone remodeling, β-TCP steadily deteriorates in animal trials before being superseded by mature fresh bone [24].

By using microtomography technique, Scarano et al. [25] determined whether micro porous tricalcium phosphate (β-TCP) and autologous platelet-derived growth agents might replace fat and hyaluronic acid, which are frequently utilized to augment the soft tissues of the oral cavity and craniofacial region in mice. The results revealed radiopaque amorphous pictures that were projected in the tender areas of each paramedian region of the right cheek, at the locations where the tricalcium phosphate/autologous platelet-derived growth agent gel had been injected. The majority of the β-TCP granules were still inside the cheek eight weeks after surgery, and were readily apparent. The edges of the β-TCP granules were distinct and did not dilute near the tissues. Tao et al. [26] in his investigation tried to improve the in vivo breakdown and bone tissue formation of β-TCP by adding PLGA and administering ASP locally in lower amounts. The results of the investigation demonstrated that bone restoration by PLGA/-TCP/ASP occurred in a dose-dependent way and that the single-dose regional application of ASP and β-TCP/PLGA had a cumulative impact on local bone creation in osteoporosis rats.

In his investigation, Huang et al. [27] uses human dental pulp cells to examine the physicochemical and biological impacts of traditional chinese medicines on the calcium silicate (CS)/tricalcium phosphate (β-TCP) nanocomposite of bone cells by synthesizing a variety of β-TCP/CS composites with varying Xu Duan (XD) ratios to create new biologically active and disposable biocomposites for rehabilitation of bones and demostrated that these calcium-based composite cements have the potential to be effective bone healing materials because of the interaction between XD in β-TCP breakdown and CS osteogenesis.

1.2.4 WHITLOCKITE

In contrast to its fabricated equivalent, β-tricalcium phosphate (β-$Ca_3(PO_4)_2$), *c* is a unique type of calcium phosphate. Additionally, WH is relatively stable in an acidic environment, unlike HAP. Due to its acidic tolerance and greater detecting in bone under higher loading, brief micro-ranged WH may serve as an inorganic blueprint element for subsequent calcification [28]. Furthermore, the higher percentage of WH in juvenile bone suggests that it may have a role in the process of bone remodeling. According to recent findings whitlockite, also known as $Ca_{18}Mg_2(HPO_4)_2(PO_4)_{12}$, is thought to be one of the primary elements of the inorganic portion of bone. Despite being a very uncommon element in the environment, WH is the second most widespread mineral in human bone, accounting for up to 20% of all bone mass, and is particularly prevalent in bone that experiences high dynamical stress [29].

In his study, Jin et al. [30] evaluated the osteoinductivity of whitlockite, hydroxyapatite, and tricalcium phosphate permeable aggregates with an SD rat spine posterolateral union model and investigated into the possibility that whitlockite could cause abnormal ossification with an SD rat abdominal pouch model. In spinal fusion, whitlockite may be an improved bone source than hydroxyapatite and tricalcium phosphate due to its reduced risk of causing abnormal ossification.

Amirthalingam et al. [31] investigated the effects of nWH/nBG and FGF-18 when administered via chitin-PLGA hydrogel to nHAP and FGF-18 and demonstrated that CGnWHF had nearly full bone regeneration, with the highest BV/TV% and synergistic effects. Overall, his study indicates that using CGnWHF to treat irregular craniofacial bone abnormalities may be a viable approach. By using simple rejuvenation chemistry Muthiah et al. [32] created an injectable 2%Ch–4%nWH hybrid hydrogel with a homogeneous dispersion of nWH. The results demonstrated that the ability of the created 2%Ch–4%nWH hybrid hydrogel to trigger the cycle of coagulation and achieve rapid and efficient hemostasis at the same time. In urgent cases, a newly created hybrid hydrogel might be able to reduce haemorrhage.

1.3 PROPERTIES OF CALCIUM PHOSPHATE

CaP is a compound that consists of calcium cations (Ca^{2+}) and phosphate anions ($PO_4{}^{3-}$). The chemical formula for calcium phosphate can vary depending on the specific compound, but the most common forms include HydroxyApatite ($Ca_5(PO_4)_3$), tricalcium phosphate ($Ca_3(PO_4)_2$), whitlockite ($Ca_9(PO_4)_6PO_3OH$), etc. CaP is biocompatible, meaning it is compatible with living tissues and can be used in biomedical applications [33]. It is commonly used as a biomaterial in bone grafting and dental applications due to its ability to support bone growth and integration with the surrounding tissues. It is a vital component of the mineralized matrix in bones and teeth. Due to its excellent mechanical properties, it provides strength and rigidity to these structures, contributing to their overall strength [34].

1.3.1 MECHANICAL PROPERTIES

Calcium phosphate, in its crystalline form, primarily hydroxyapatite, exhibits several mechanical properties that contribute to its role in providing strength and rigidity to bones and teeth. CaP possesses remarkable compressive strength, enabling it to withstand significant loads without fracturing [35]. This property is particularly important in load-bearing applications such as dental implants and orthopedic implants, where the material must support the weight and forces exerted on it. These properties make it a highly desirable material in various biomedical applications [36].

1.3.1.1 Hardness

Hardness refers to a material's resistance to indentation, scratching, or deformation. The hardness of CaP compounds can vary depending on their specific composition and crystal structure [39]. In general, CaP materials used in biomedical applications have hardness values similar to natural bone. The hardness of natural bone can vary, but it typically falls within the range of 2–5 on the Mohr's scale [40]. Therefore, CaP

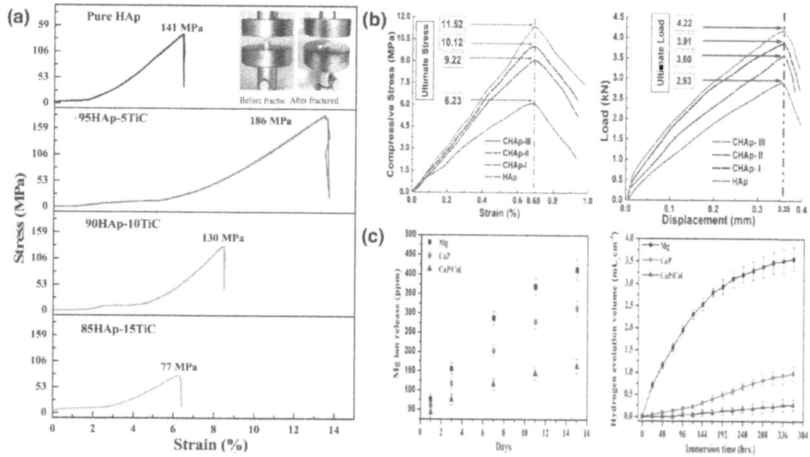

Figure 1.3 (a) Mechanical behavior of prepared samples with different composition of HAp and TiC [45]. (Reprinted from Avinashi *et al.* Copyrights Elsevier 2022.) (b) Difference in compressive strength and fracture toughness property with change in carbonate content [16]. (Reprinted from Bhatnagar *et al.* Copyrights Elsevier 2023.) (c) Mg-ion release rate and Hydrogen evolution rate of prepared samples when immersed in SBF solution depicting corrosion behavior of synthesized samples [38]. (Reprinted from Guo *et al.* Copyrights Elsevier 2020.)

materials used for biomedical purposes, such as hydroxyapatite coatings on orthopedic implants or bone graft substitutes, are designed to have a similar hardness to natural bone to facilitate integration and minimize stress-shielding effects.

Baradaran et al. [37] synthesized hydroxyapatite and Ni-doped HAp mixed with graphene nanoplatelets to evaluate mechanical and biological properties. The samples were synthesized using a continuous precipitation method and then calcined at 900 °C for 1 h. Then, graphene was reinforced in the sample using rotary ball milling technique. The results demonstrated the rise in hardness and mechanical behavior in samples with an increase in doping as shown in Figure 1.3(a). Hardness increases by 55%–75% due to Ni-doping and incorporation of graphene nanoplatelets.

Aarthy et al. [41] naturally derive the calcium phosphate i.e., from the goat bone. The influence of the sintering temperature on the naturally derived biomaterial on mechanical and biological properties has been evaluated. First, the clean goat bones were collected and boiled as well as treated with 2M NaOH for 6 hours. Then, the obtained sample was washed and dried at 100 °C for 24 hours. Furthermore, it is calcined at 900 °C and ball milled for further treatment. Then, the samples were sintered at 1100, 1200, 1300, and 1400 °C. The results demonstrated the increase in hardness with a rise in temperature. The sample sintered at 1400 °C shows the maximum hardness i.e., 301.3 MPa. It was concluded that it can also influence the hardness using sintering at different temperatures and naturally derived calcium phosphate can find better applications than chemically derived samples.

Overall, the hardness of calcium phosphate materials for biomedical applications is typically tailored to closely match the hardness of natural bone to ensure compatibility and promote successful integration within the body.

1.3.1.2 Fracture Toughness

Fracture toughness is an important mechanical property that measures a material's resistance to crack propagation. However, the fracture toughness of calcium phosphate materials can vary depending on the specific composition, processing method, and testing conditions [42]. CaP materials, such as hydroxyapatite (HAp) and tricalcium phosphate (TCP), generally exhibit lower fracture toughness compared to natural bone [43]. The fracture toughness values for these materials typically range from 1 to 3 MPa/m, which is considerably lower than the values observed for metals or tougher ceramics [44]. In load-bearing situations, they are often combined with tougher materials or reinforced with fibers or other additives to enhance their overall mechanical performance.

Avinashi et al. [45] synthesized hydroxyapatite (HAp) and titanium carbide (TiC) doped HAp samples a wet chemical precipitation method and a solid-state reaction method, respectively. Four different samples with varying compositions of TiC were prepared to evaluate mechanical properties. The results revealed the ultimate compressive strength and fracture toughness was found to be maximum for 5 wt% of TiC in composite sample. Further increasing the concentration of TiC lead to decrease in strength and fracture toughness property. Samples containing 5 wt% TiC was found to be mechanically best.

Bhatnagar et al. [16] synthesized carbonate doped hydroxyapatite samples using hydrothermal synthesis technique. Samples with different stoichiometric compositions was synthesized for structural and mechanical analysis. The results demonstrated the increase in compressive strength as well as fracture toughness with an increase in carbonate composition in the samples. Figure 1.3(b) depicts that the sample containing 15 wt% of carbonate (CO_3^{2-}) showed the highest fracture toughness. It was concluded that carbonate doped HAp can be used to develop bone cement and also as a coating on bio-implant due to its mechanically stable characteristic.

It's worth noting that the mechanical properties of calcium phosphate can vary depending on factors such as crystalline structure, composition, porosity, and processing methods. Additionally, the mechanical properties of bone, which consist of a composite of calcium phosphate and organic materials, are also influenced by the overall structure and organization of the bone tissue.

1.3.2 BIOLOGICAL PROPERTIES

CaP possesses remarkable biological properties that make it highly suitable for medical applications. Its excellent biocompatibility ensures compatibility with living tissues, minimizing the risk of rejection or adverse reactions [46]. As an osteoconductive material, it promotes bone growth and regeneration, enabling the integration of the implant with surrounding bone. The bioactivity of CaP facilitates chemical bonding with bone tissue, enhancing the stability and longevity of the implant through osseointegration [47]. Additionally, its controlled resorption allows for gradual replacement by natural bone, facilitating long-term healing. Furthermore, its radiopacity enables easy monitoring and assessment of implant positioning and integration using medical imaging techniques. These inherent biological properties make calcium phosphate an invaluable material for a wide range of medical applications, such as bone grafts, dental implants, and orthopedic devices [48].

1.3.2.1 Biodegradability

One of the important properties of CaP in biomedical applications is its biodegradability. Biodegradability refers to the ability of a material to undergo degradation or breakdown by natural biological processes over time [49]. CaP, particularly in certain forms such as tricalcium phosphate (TCP) and dicalcium phosphate dihydrate (DCPD), exhibits biodegradable characteristics. When used in biomedical implants, calcium phosphate materials gradually degrade and are resorbed by the body's natural processes [50,51]. As new bone tissue forms and integrates with the implant, the calcium phosphate undergoes a gradual breakdown, allowing the body to replace it with natural bone over time. This process is known as biodegradation or bioresorption.

Guo et al. [38] prepared composite coating of calcium phosphate and collagen and then successfully fabricated on the surface of magnesium alloy. The coatings were fabricated on the surface using dip coating technique. The degradability and corrosion resistance property was investigated using electrochemical and immersion tests. The immersion test in SBF solution results present in Figure 1.3(c) demonstrates the enhancement in corrosion resistance due to inclusion of collagen and CaP coating. These observations are very promising and it was concluded that CaP/Col coating could definitely protect Mg alloy from further degradation, thus making it a great candidate for implant applications.

The rate of biodegradation of calcium phosphate can be controlled by adjusting factors such as composition, crystallinity, and porosity of the material. By modifying these parameters, the degradation rate can be tailored to match the desired healing timeline of the specific implant application.

1.3.2.2 Biocompatibility

Calcium phosphate demonstrates exceptional biocompatibility, making it a highly sought-after material in the field of biomedicine. When in contact with living tissues, calcium phosphate materials elicit minimal adverse reactions or cytotoxic effects [53,54]. This property ensures that they are well-tolerated by the body, reducing the risk of inflammation or immune response. CaP exhibits compatibility with various tissues, including bone, teeth, and soft tissues, enabling its use in a wide range of biomedical applications [55]. Cells readily interact with CaP, attaching, spreading, and proliferating on its surface, promoting tissue regeneration and integration.

Gao et al. [52] synthesized the CaP material and then deposited the coating on magnesium alloy using chemical conversion method. The biodegradation and

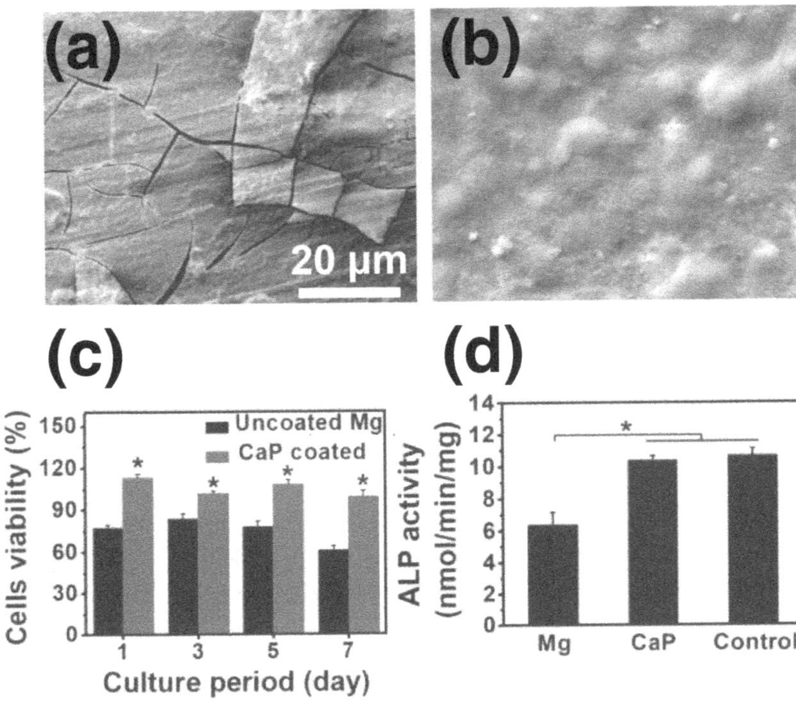

Figure 1.4 Morphology of MC3T3-E1 cells when cultured on (a) uncoated, (b) Calicum Phosphate coated samples, (c) cell viability, and (d) ALP activity when cells cultured with extracts of prepare samples by Gao *et al.* [52].

biocompatibility properties were evaluated and compared with uncoated Mg alloy. The results revealed better cell behavior, cell proliferation and cell adhesion due to CaP coating. The in-vivo and in-vitro both the tests showed better biocompatible behavior than uncoated Mg alloy as depicted in Figure 1.4(a–d). It was concluded that CaP coating can significantly improve the biocompatibility behavior of bio-implants.

Overall, the biocompatibility of calcium phosphate is a critical factor that contributes to its wide usage in biomedical applications, including bone grafts, dental implants, coatings for implants, and tissue engineering scaffolds. The compatibility with host tissues and the ability to support cell viability, mineralization, and tissue regeneration make calcium phosphate an ideal biomaterial in various clinical scenarios.

1.4 TOXICITY ASSESSMENT

Toxicity assessment of calcium phosphate involves evaluating its potential adverse effects based on factors such as its chemical composition, physical form, dosage, route of exposure, and duration of exposure [57]. Toxicity assessments require comprehensive and rigorous scientific studies, including in vitro experiments, animal studies, and human clinical trials. These studies help determine the potential risks associated with calcium phosphate exposure. Generally, calcium phosphate is considered to have low toxicity but exposure to high concentration can still lead to deadly infection and diseases [58].

By using chemical conversion technique Guo et al. [59] created a CaP wrapping with a micro-nanofibrous porosity framework on the exposed outer layer of the magnesium alloy and demonstrated that the CaP coating exhibited outstanding biological compatibility, which could successfully enhance the proliferation, and attachment of osteoblasts, with the aid of a thorough assessment of cell sustainability, ALP activity, and cell shapes and concluded that the CaP coating shows significant promise for the development of disposable Mg-based orthopaedic implant devices.

In his work, Akram et al. [60] developed chitosan (CCP) diffused hemostatic dressing materials with calcium phosphate nanoflakes (CaP-NFs). A variety of biochemical tests were run to determine the effectiveness of the CCP-based hemostatic dressing materials. Additionally, both gram-positive and gram-negative isolates of bacteria were used to test the dressing materials and concluded that CCP-based hemostatic dressing materials are extremely biocompatible and immediately promoted blood to coagulate under 15 seconds of exposure.

The functionally scaled biomaterials of calcium phosphate/titanium alloys were cast using a novel process by El et al. [56]. While whitlockite ($Ca_3(PO_4)_2$) was produced in the context of the Ti6Al-4V alloy, $CaHPO_4$ served as the calcium-containing component in the Ti-6Al-7Nb alloy. After casting, the samples were ready for testing osseointegration, in-vivo systemic toxicity, and in-vitro cytocompatibility. The cell viability results and analysis of H&E dyed dog's jaw bones shown in Figure 1.5(a,b) revealed that as compared to Ti-6Al-4V FGBMs, the Ti-6Al-7Nb FGBMs has better survival of cells and a satisfactory cytocompatibility.

In his study Le et al. [53] looked at two calcium-phosphate (CaP)-based composites biological compatibility and osteoinductive abilities both in vitro and in vivo. When the biocompatibility of the pellets was assessed in vitro using osteoblast-like MG-63 cells, the cell shape and proliferation revealed identical initial behavior. In a cranial rat model, freshly produced bone and the ability to degrade of the investigational constructs were assessed for in vivo biocompatibility and concluded that both HA and HA-TCP scaffolds produced using the SLA 3D printing approach are cytocompatible and enable in vivo bone regeneration in a rat osteo enhancement model without the presence of any severe inflammatory reactions.

In his study, Meng et al. [61] assessed in vitro and vivo biological compatibility of a pair of new injectable, biologically active cements: chitosan microsphere/CPC and β-tricalcium phosphate (β-TCP)/CPC. The in vitro cell investigation revealed good biocompatibility and concluded that chitosan microsphere/CPC and β-TCP/CPC composites could be effective injectable materials for repairing damaged bone.

Its particle size and solubility can influence the toxicity of calcium phosphate. Fine particles or nanoparticles of calcium phosphate may have unique properties and

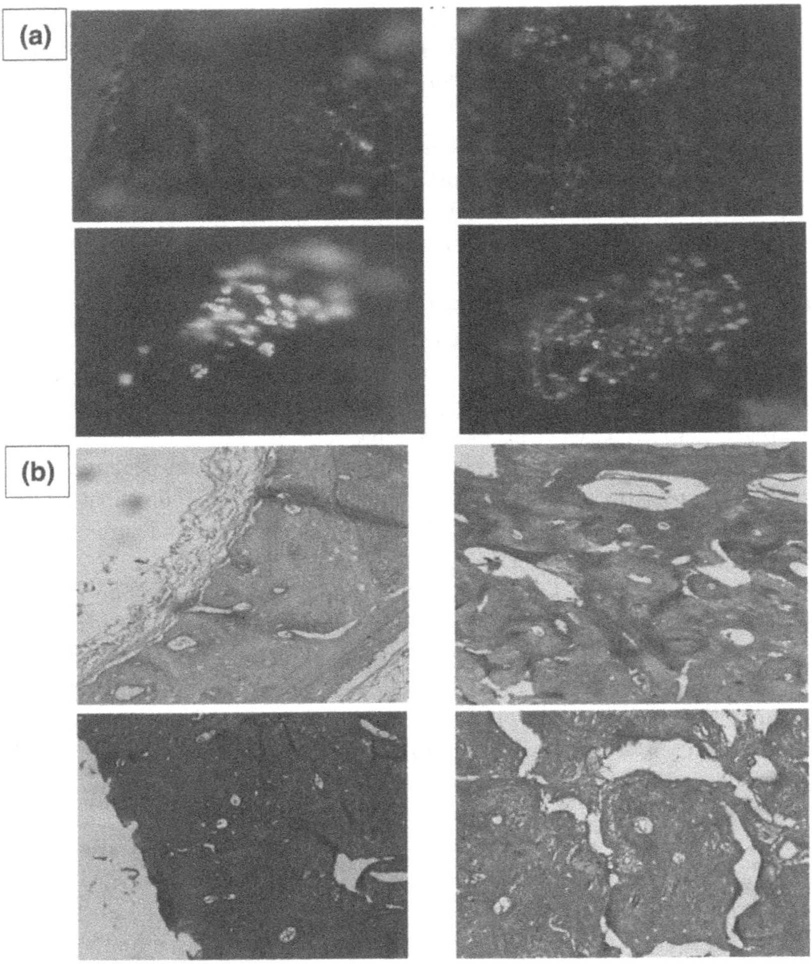

Figure 1.5 (a) Illustration depicting surface interaction of cells and implant with each other when stained with AO/EB when analyzed under fluorescence microscope, where green color represents live cells and orange stain is used for dead cells. (b) Images representing H & E dyed bone slides of dog's jaw bones when analyzed under an electronic microscope with 200× magnification [56]. (Reprinted from El *et al.* Copyrights Elsevier 2018.)

potentially greater toxicity compared to larger particles. In general, CaP is biocompatible and non-toxic as it is found naturally in the human body.

1.5 FUTURE PERSPECTIVE AND CONCLUSION

The fields of tissue engineering, regenerative medicine, drug delivery systems, and bioactive coatings have all showed tremendous prospects for CaP-based materials.

Prospective research and advancement of diverse biomedical uses will determine how biocompatible CaP is. The characteristics of CaP materials are anticipated to be optimized in the upcoming years in order to further increase their biocompatibility. In order to more closely resemble the external medium found in living things and encourage cell adhesion, proliferation, and differentiation, it may be necessary to alter the composition, morphology, surface qualities, and mechanical characteristics of these materials. Advances in nanotechnology might make it possible to create brand-new calcium phosphate materials with innovative nanostructures that are more biocompatible. Enhanced biocompatibility and tissue regeneration may be provided by nanoscale properties, including increased surface area and enhanced cellular contact. Investigations may be based upon looking into adding stem cells, bioactive compounds, and growth factors to calcium phosphate-based polymers to increase their capacity for regeneration. This might result in the creation of bioactive scaffolds that actively encourage tissue growth and regeneration as well as structural support.

In conclusion, CaP's biocompatibility has already demonstrated its potential in a number of biological applications. We may anticipate future developments in improving the biocompatibility of CaP materials as research and development in the area continues. These developments will help create creative and practical approaches for tissue engineering, regenerative medicine, and other biomedical applications, ultimately enhancing patient outcomes and quality of life.

REFERENCES

1. T. Biswal, S. Kumar BadJena, and D. Pradhan. Sustainable biomaterials and their applications: A short review. *Materials Today*, **30**:274–282, 2020.
2. L. F. Santos, I. J. Correia, A. S. Silva, and J. F. Mano. Biomaterials for drug delivery patches. *European Journal of Pharmaceutical Sciences*, **118**:49–66, 2018.
3. S. Gautam, D. Bhatnagar, D. Bansal, H. Batra, and N. Goyal. Recent advancements in nanomaterials for biomedical implants. *Biomedical Engineering Advances*, **1**:100029, 2022.
4. S. Gautam, D. Bansal, D. Bhatnagar, C. Sharma, and N. Goyal. Synthesis of iron-based nanoparticles by chemical methods and their biomedical applications. In *Oxides for Medical Applications*, pp. 167–195. Elsevier, 2023.
5. S. Basu and B. Basu. Unravelling doped biphasic calcium phosphate: Synthesis to application. *ACS Applied Bio Materials*, **2**(12):5263–5297, 2019.
6. N. W. Kucko, R.-P. Herber, S. C. G. Leeuwenburgh, and J. A. Jansen. Calcium phosphate bioceramics and cements. In *Principles of Regenerative Medicine*, pp. 591–611. Elsevier, 2019.
7. M. A. Sakr, K. Sakthivel, T. Hossain, S. R. Shin, S. Siddiqua, J. Kim, and K. Kim. Recent trends in gelatin methacryloyl nanocomposite hydrogels for tissue engineering. *Journal of Biomedical Materials Research Part A*, **110**(3):708–724, 2022.
8. N. Eliaz and N. Metoki. Calcium phosphate bioceramics: A review of their history, structure, properties, coating technologies and biomedical applications. *Materials*, **10**(4):334, 2017.
9. I. El Bialy, W. Jiskoot, and M. R. Nejadnik. Formulation, delivery and stability of bone morphogenetic proteins for effective bone regeneration. *Pharmaceutical Research*, **34**:1152–1170, 2017.

10. C. Sharma, D. Bansal, D. Bhatnagar, S. Gautam, and N. Goyal. Advanced nanomaterials: From properties and perspective applications to their interlinked confronts. In *Advanced Functional Nanoparticles "Boon or Bane" for Environment Remediation Applications: Combating Environmental Issues*, pp. 1–6. Springer, 2023.
11. D. Bansal, D. Bhatnagar, D. Rana, and S. Gautam. Ferrite nanoparticles in food technology. In *Applications of Nanostructured Ferrites*, pp. 295–314. Elsevier, 2023.
12. L.-H. Fu, Y.-R. Hu, C. Qi, T. He, S. Jiang, C. Jiang, J. He, J. Qu, J. Lin, and P. Huang. Biodegradable manganese-doped calcium phosphate nanotheranostics for traceable cascade reaction-enhanced anti-tumor therapy. *Acs Nano*, **13**(12):13985–13994, 2019.
13. R. Kamphof, R. N. Lima, J. W. Schoones, J. J. Arts, R. G. Nelissen, G. Cama, and B. G. Pijls. Antimicrobial activity of ion-substituted calcium phosphates: A systematic review. *Heliyon*, 2023.
14. D. Xiao, J. Zhang, C. Zhang, D. Barbieri, H. Yuan, L. Moroni, and G. Feng. The role of calcium phosphate surface structure in osteogenesis and the mechanisms involved. *Acta Biomaterialia*, **106**:22–33, 2020.
15. B. Priyadarshini, M. Rama, Chetan, and U. Vijayalakshmi. Bioactive coating as a surface modification technique for biocompatible metallic implants: A review. *Journal of Asian Ceramic Societies*, **7**(4):397–406, 2019.
16. D. Bhatnagar, S. Gautam, H. Batra, and N. Goyal. Enhancement of fracture toughness in carbonate doped hydroxyapatite based nanocomposites: Rietveld analysis and mechanical behaviour. *Journal of the Mechanical Behavior of Biomedical Materials*, **142**:105814, 2023.
17. H. Shao, J. He, T. Lin, Z. Zhang, Y. Zhang, and S. Liu. 3D gel-printing of hydroxyapatite scaffold for bone tissue engineering. *Ceramics International*, **45**(1):1163–1170, 2019.
18. B. Ren, X. Chen, S. Du, Y. Ma, H. Chen, G. Yuan, J. Li, D. Xiong, H. Tan, Z. Ling, Y. Chen, X. Hu, and X. Niu. Injectable polysaccharide hydrogel embedded with hydroxyapatite and calcium carbonate for drug delivery and bone tissue engineering. *International Journal of Biological Macromolecules*, **118**:1257–1266, 2018.
19. A. A. Mirtchi, J. Lemaitre, and N. Terao. Calcium phosphate cements: Study of the β-tricalcium phosphate–monocalcium phosphate system. *Biomaterials*, **10**(7):475–480, 1989.
20. K Hurle, J. M. Oliveira, R. L. Reis, S. Pina, and F. Goetz-Neunhoeffer. Ion-doped brushite cements for bone regeneration. *Acta Biomaterialia*, **123**:51–71, 2021.
21. Y. Zhuang, Q. Liu, G. Jia, H. Li, G. Yuan, and H. Yu. A biomimetic zinc alloy scaffold coated with brushite for enhanced cranial bone regeneration. *ACS Biomaterials Science & Engineering*, **7**(3):893–903, 2020.
22. N. Sudhan, S. Anitta, S. Meenakshi, and C. Sekar. Brushite nanoparticles based electrochemical sensor for detection of uric acid, xanthine, hypoxanthine and caffeine. *Analytical Biochemistry*, **659**:114947, 2022.
23. M. Rödel, J. Tesmar, J. Groll, and U. Gbureck. Dual setting brushite–gelatin cement with increased ductility and sustained drug release. *Journal of Biomaterials Applications*, **36**(10):1882–1898, 2022.
24. N. Kabilan, N. Karthikeyan, K. D. Babu, and K. Chinnakali. Third-order nonlinear optical properties of mono and biphasic β-tricalcium phosphate in continuous wave regime. *Journal of Materials Science: Materials in Electronics*, **34**(10):1–2, 2023.
25. A. Scarano, L. Valbonetti, M. Marchetti, F. Lorusso, and M. Ceccarelli. Soft tissue augmentation of the face with autologous platelet-derived growth factors and tricalcium phosphate. Microtomography evaluation of mice. *Journal of Craniofacial Surgery*, **27**(5):1212–1214, 2016.

26. Z.-S. Tao, X.-J. Wu, W.-S. Zhou, X.-Ju Wu, W. Liao, M. Yang, H.-G. Xu, and L. Yang. Local administration of aspirin with β-tricalcium phosphate/poly-lactic-coglycolic acid (β-tcp/plga) could enhance osteoporotic bone regeneration. *Journal of Bone and Mineral Metabolism*, **37**:1026–035, 2019.
27. M.-H. Huang, C.-T. Kao, Y.-W. Chen, T.-T. Hsu, D.-E. Shieh, T.-H. Huang, and M.-Y. Shie. The synergistic effects of Chinese herb and injectable calcium silicate/β-tricalcium phosphate composite on an osteogenic accelerator in vitro. *Journal of Materials Science: Materials in Medicine*, **26**:1–2, 2015.
28. R. Lagier and C.-A. Baud. Magnesium whitlockite, a calcium phosphate crystal of special interest in pathology. *Pathology-Research and Practice*, **199**(5):329–335, 2003.
29. H. D. Kim, H. L. Jang, H.-Y. Ahn, H. K. Lee, J. Park, E.-S. Lee, E. A. Lee, Y.-H. Jeong, D.-G. Kim, K. T. Nam, and N. S. Hwang. Biomimetic whitlockite inorganic nanoparticles-mediated in situ remodeling and rapid bone regeneration. *Biomaterials*, **112**:31–43, 2017.
30. Y.-Z. Jin, G.-B. Zheng, M. Cho, and J. H. Lee. Effect of whitlockite as a new bone substitute for bone formation in spinal fusion and ectopic ossification animal model. *Biomaterials Research*, **25**(1):1–7, 2021.
31. S. Amirthalingam, S. S. Lee, M. Pandian, J. Ramu, S. Iyer, N. S. Hwang, and R. Jayakumar. Combinatorial effect of nano whitlockite/nano bioglass with FGF-18 in an injectable hydrogel for craniofacial bone regeneration. *Biomaterials Science*, **9**(7):2439–2453, 2021.
32. N. S. M. Pillai, K. Eswar, S. Amirthalingam, U. Mony, P. K. Varma, and R. Jayakumar. Injectable nano whitlockite incorporated chitosan hydrogel for effective hemostasis. *ACS Applied Bio Materials*, **2**(2):865–873, 2019.
33. H. H. K. Xu, P. Wang, L. Wang, C. Bao, Q. Chen, M. D. Weir, L. C. Chow, L. Zhao, X. Zhou, and M. A. Reynolds. Calcium phosphate cements for bone engineering and their biological properties. *Bone Research*, **5**(1):1–19, 2017.
34. R. O'neill, H. O. McCarthy, E. B. Montufar, M.-P. Ginebra, D. I. Wilson, A. Lennon, and N. Dunne. Critical review: Injectability of calcium phosphate pastes and cements. *Acta Biomaterialia*, **50**:1–9, 2017.
35. Q. Li, C. Feng, Q. Cao, W. Wang, Z. Ma, Y. Wu, T. He, Y. Jing, W. Tan, T. Liao, J. Xing, and X. Li. Strategies of strengthening mechanical properties in the osteoinductive calcium phosphate bioceramics. *Regenerative Biomaterials*, **10**:rbad013, 2023.
36. F. Hajiali, S. Tajbakhsh, and A. Shojaei. Fabrication and properties of polycaprolactone composites containing calcium phosphate-based ceramics and bioactive glasses in bone tissue engineering: A review. *Polymer Reviews*, **58**(1):164–207, 2018.
37. S. Baradaran, E. Moghaddam, B. Nasiri-Tabrizi, W. J. Basirun, M. Mehrali, M. H. Sookhakian, and Y. Alias. Characterization of nickel-doped biphasic calcium phosphate/graphene nanoplatelet composites for biomedical application. *Materials Science and Engineering: C*, **49**:656–668, 2015.
38. Y. Guo, Y. Su, R. Gu, Z. Zhang, G. Li, J. Lian, and L. Ren. Enhanced corrosion resistance and biocompatibility of biodegradable magnesium alloy modified by calcium phosphate/collagen coating. *Surface and Coatings Technology*, **401**:126318, 2020.
39. Z. Dai, X. Xie, N. Zhang, S. Li, K. Yang, M. Zhu, M. D. Weir, H. H. K. Xu, K. Zhang, Z. Zhao, and Y. Bai. Novel nanostructured resin infiltrant containing calcium phosphate nanoparticles to prevent enamel white spot lesions. *Journal of the Mechanical Behavior of Biomedical Materials*, **126**:104990, 2022.

40. Z. Okulus and A. Voelkel. Mechanical properties of experimental composites with different calcium phosphates fillers. *Materials Science and Engineering: C*, **78**:1101–1108, 2017.
41. S. Aarthy, D. Thenmuhil, G. Dharunya, and P. Manohar. Exploring the effect of sintering temperature on naturally derived hydroxyapatite for bio-medical applications. *Journal of Materials Science: Materials in Medicine*, **30**:1–11, 2019.
42. L. Sun and D. Guo. Study on the improvement of compressive strength and fracture toughness of calcium phosphate cement. *Ceramics International*, **48**(13):18579–18587, 2022.
43. P. Dee, H. Y. You, S.-H. Teoh, and H. L. Ferrand. Bioinspired approaches to toughen calcium phosphate-based ceramics for bone repair. *Journal of the Mechanical Behavior of Biomedical Materials*, **112**:104078, 2020.
44. Y. Wang, M. Wang, F. Chen, C. Feng, X. Chen, X. Li, Y. Xiao, and X. Zhang. Enhancing mechanical and biological properties of biphasic calcium phosphate ceramics by adding calcium oxide. *Journal of the American Ceramic Society*, **104**(1):548–563, 2021.
45. S. K. Avinashi, P. Singh, K. Sharma, A. Hussain, D. Singh, and C. Gautam. Morphological, mechanical, and biological evolution of pure hydroxyapatite and its composites with titanium carbide for biomedical applications. *Ceramics International*, **48**(13):18475–18489, 2022.
46. J. Lu, H. Yu, and C. Chen. Biological properties of calcium phosphate biomaterials for bone repair: A review. *RSC Advances*, **8**(4):2015–2033, 2018.
47. Z. Yuan, J. Bi, W. Wang, X. Sun, L. Wang, J. Mao, and F. Yang. A novel synthesis method and properties of calcium-deficient hydroxyapatite/α-TCP biphasic calcium phosphate. *Journal of Biomaterials Applications*, **36**(9):1712–1719, 2022.
48. Q. Zhang, Z. Lei, M. Peng, M. Zhong, Y. Wan, and H. Luo. Enhancement of mechanical and biological properties of calcium phosphate bone cement by incorporating bacterial cellulose. *Materials Technology*, **34**(13):800–806, 2019.
49. I. Lodoso-Torrecilla, J. J. J. P. van den Beucken, and J. A. Jansen. Calcium phosphate cements: Optimization toward biodegradability. *Acta Biomaterialia*, **119**:1–12, 2021.
50. O. Suzuki, Y. Shiwaku, and R. Hamai. Octacalcium phosphate bone substitute materials: Comparison between properties of biomaterials and other calcium phosphate materials. *Dental Materials Journal*, **39**(2):187–199, 2020.
51. P. Makkar, H. J. Kang, A. R. Padalhin, O. Faruq, and B. Lee. In-vitro and in-vivo evaluation of strontium doped calcium phosphate coatings on biodegradable magnesium alloy for bone applications. *Applied Surface Science*, **510**:145333, 2020.
52. J. Gao, Y. Su, and Y.-X. Qin. Calcium phosphate coatings enhance biocompatibility and degradation resistance of magnesium alloy: Correlating in vitro and in vivo studies. *Bioactive Materials*, **6**(5):1223–1229, 2021.
53. L. L. Guéhennec, D. V. Hede, E. Plougonven, G. Nolens, B. Verlée, M.-C. De Pauw, and F. Lambert. In vitro and in vivo biocompatibility of calciumphosphate scaffolds three-dimensional printed by stereolithography for bone regeneration. *Journal of Biomedical Materials Research Part A*, **108**(3):412–425, 2020.
54. S. Mofakhami and E. Salahinejad. Biphasic calcium phosphate microspheres in biomedical applications. *Journal of Controlled Release*, **338**:527–536, 2021.
55. Y. Su, I. Cockerill, Y. Zheng, L. Tang, Y.-X. Qin, and D. Zhu. Biofunctionalization of metallic implants by calcium phosphate coatings. *Bioactive Materials*, **4**:196–206, 2019.

56. S. El-Hadad, E. M. Safwat, and N. F. Sharaf. In-vitro and in-vivo, cytotoxicity evaluation of cast functionally graded biomaterials for dental implantology. *Materials Science and Engineering: C*, **93**:987–995, 2018.
57. M. Maillard, O. N. Bandiaky, S. Maunoury, C. Alliot, B. Alliot-Licht, S. Serisier, and E. Renard. The effectiveness of calcium phosphates in the treatment of dentinal hypersensitivity: A systematic review. *Bioengineering*, **10**(4):447, 2023.
58. S. Sauro, G. Spagnuolo, C. D. Giudice, D. M. A. Neto, P. B. A. Fechine, X. Chen, S. Rengo, X. Chen, and V. P. Feitosa. Chemical, structural and cytotoxicity characterisation of experimental fluoride-doped calcium phosphates as promising remineralising materials for dental applications. *Dental Materials*, **39**(4):391–401, 2023.
59. Y. Guo, G. Li, Z. Xu, Y. Xu, L. Yin, Z. Yu, Z. Zhang, J. Lian, and L. Ren. Corrosion resistance and biocompatibility of calcium phosphate coatings with a micro–nanofibrous porous structure on biodegradable magnesium alloys. *ACS Applied Bio Materials*, **5**(4):1528–1537, 2022.
60. A. Md. Akram, R. A. Omar, and Md. Ashfaq. Chitosan/calcium phosphate-nanoflakes-based biomaterial: A potential hemostatic wound dressing material. *Polymer Bulletin*, **80**(5):5071–5086, 2023.
61. D. Meng, L. Dong, Y. Yuan, and Q. Jiang. In vitro and in vivo analysis of the biocompatibility of two novel and injectable calcium phosphate cements. *Regenerative Biomaterials*, **6**(1):13–19, 2019.

2 History of Calcium Phosphate in Regenerative Medicine

Lidiya Sonowal and Sanjeev Gautam
Advanced Functional Materials Laboratory, Dr. S.S. Bhatnagar University Institute of Chemical Engineering and Technology, Panjab University, Chandigarh, India

2.1 INTRODUCTION

By utilizing the body's innate healing mechanisms, the discipline of medicine known as regenerative medicine has the potential to completely transform healthcare. For patients with chronic illnesses, wounds, or congenital problems, this multidisciplinary approach offers new hope by attempting to repair, swap out, or regenerate damaged tissues and organs [1]. Regenerative medicine aims to activate the body's natural repair mechanisms to enhance healing and functional recovery through the use of stem cells, tissue engineering, gene therapy, and other cutting-edge methods. Stem cells play a pivotal role in regenerative medicine, as they possess the remarkable ability to differentiate into various specialized cell types [2]. Tissue engineering is another vital component of regenerative medicine, involving the fabrication of artificial tissues and organs using a combination of cells, biomaterials, and biochemical factors [3]. Gene therapy, on the other hand, focuses on correcting genetic defects responsible for certain diseases by introducing therapeutic genes into a patient's cells [4].

Besides bone tissue engineering, calcium phosphate has more recently been used in regenerative medicine. Its potential in other regenerative medicine fields, like cartilage regeneration and wound healing, is being investigated by researchers. Calcium phosphate materials have demonstrated potential in boosting chondrogenic differentiation and encouraging the development of new cartilage-like tissue when utilized in cartilage repair. This is crucial for diseases like osteoarthritis, which cause cartilage deterioration and injury [5]. Additionally, calcium phosphate-based substances have been used to create bioactive coatings for implants. These coatings improve the fusion of medical devices' surfaces with surrounding tissues, lowering the chance of

DOI: 10.1201/9781003360605-2

implant rejection and enhancing long-term stability, such as orthopaedic implants or dental fixtures [6].

Calcium phosphate dressings have been studied in the area of wound healing for their potential to encourage tissue regeneration and hasten the healing process. These dressings aid in wound closure while also providing an environment that is favorable for cell migration and tissue growth [7]. Continuous research attempts to enhance the characteristics of calcium phosphate materials, create new formulations, and investigate fresh uses as they continue to show their versatility and potential in regenerative medicine. However, there is still much to learn about issues like regulating scaffold degradation rates, making sure that bioactive molecule release is precisely controlled, and dealing with potential immunological reactions [8].

Overall, the use of calcium phosphate in regenerative medicine has enormous potential to advance medical procedures and enhance the lives of patients with varied tissue and organ abnormalities. We may anticipate even more ground-breaking advancements in the field of regenerative medicine as technology and our understanding of these materials grow. These breakthroughs will offer up new possibilities for therapeutic interventions and tissue restoration.

2.2 EARLY DISCOVERIES AND RECOGNITION

The natural mending of bone injuries was well understood by ancient cultures, revealing an early awareness of bone healing even before current medical developments. All of these societies, including Mesoamerica, India, China, and ancient Egypt, have in-depth observations and remedies for bone fractures and wounds [9]. Ancient healers and physicians played important roles in their communities and were highly regarded for their knowledge of bone mending. They frequently preserved and disseminated their medical insights across generations by passing on their knowledge through oral traditions, apprenticeships, and written documents [10]. In ancient times, the idea of bone healing was inextricably linked to spiritual and religious beliefs. A belief in the interdependence of the body, mind, and spirit in the healing process is shown in the widespread performance of healing rituals and prayers alongside medical treatments. These all-encompassing methods of bone healing stressed the significance of not only physical health but also mental and spiritual health [11]. The ancient civilizations' inventiveness and comprehension of the therapeutic capabilities of the environment is demonstrated by their use of natural substances, such as plants, herbs, and animal products, for bone mending. Many of these conventional treatments have now been researched and used as important sources of therapeutic chemicals in contemporary medicine [12]. Ancient understanding of bone healing also played a role in the creation of medical systems and traditions that still have an impact on modern healthcare practises. Ancient medical theories that lay the foundation for the development of orthopaedics include knowledge of bone structure, the value of immobilization, and the use of traction [13]. Modern orthopaedics improves on the foundation laid down by ancient civilizations by utilizing cutting-edge imaging technologies, surgical procedures, and medical equipment. The diagnosis,

Table 2.1
Notable Pioneers and Their Contribution in the Field of Regenerative Medicines

Pioneers	Investigation	Demonstrations	References
Marshall R. Urist	Bone Morphogenetic Proteins (BMPs)	Discovered that BMPs were powerful bone-inducing agents leading to the creation of artificial bone substitutes	[15]
Per-Ingvar Brånemark	Osseointegration	Developed the idea to osseointegrated implants for several orthopaedic uses	[16]
Dr. Larry L. Hench	Calcium Phosphate Cement	Use of CPC as a synthetic biomaterial for bone void filling	[17]
Dr. Arnold Caplan	Mesenchymal Stem Cells	Coining the term "mesenchymal stem cells" and illustrated their use in regenerative medicines	[18]

management, and treatment of bone injuries in modern medicine are still shaped by the information accumulated over centuries of observations and interventions [14].

Orthopaedic surgery and regenerative medicine have advanced significantly because of ground-breaking researchers in bone graft alternatives. These pioneers have committed their work to creating and researching cutting-edge materials and procedures that can supplement or replace natural bone transplants.

Some of the notable pioneers and their contributions are being summarized in Table 2.1

2.3 ADVANCEMENTS IN BIOACTIVITY

In the areas of biomaterials and tissue engineering, improvements in the bioactivity of calcium phosphate have been a key subject of research and development. Tricalcium phosphate (TCP) and hydroxyapatite (HA), two calcium phosphate compounds, are particularly well suited for use in bone repair and regeneration because of their biocompatibility and capacity to imitate the mineral makeup of real bone [19, 20]. This section attempts to discuss the bioactive nature of calcium phosphate and its interaction with living tissues in brief. Figure 2.1 illustrates the key words associated with bioactivity of calcium phosphate.

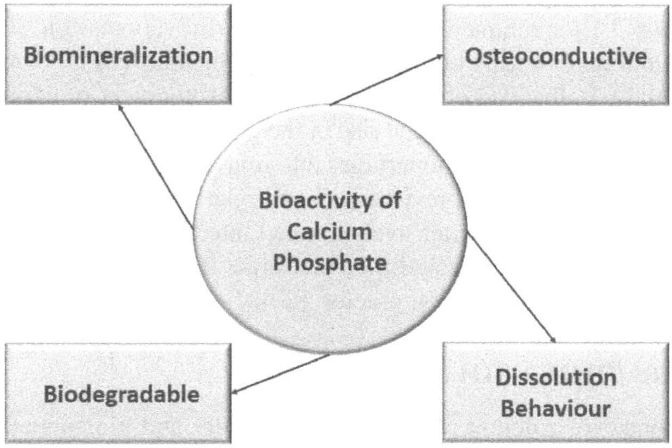

Figure 2.1 Keywords associated with bioactivity of calcium phosphate in regenerative medicine.

2.3.1 BIOACTIVE NATURE OF CALCIUM PHOSPHATE

Calcium phosphate's bioactivity originates from its particular capacity to interact positively with biological systems and living tissues. Due to this quality, it is a highly sought-after substance in the fields of biomedical engineering and regenerative medicine [21]. Its ability to promote biomineralization is one of the primary characteristics that contributes to its bioactivity. Calcium phosphate starts the deposition of calcium and phosphate ions on its surface when it comes into touch with biological fluids or tissues, which results in the creation of an apatite layer that resembles bone. This apatite production supports the development of new bone cells and allows for smooth interaction with surrounding tissues. Further, the exceptional osteoconductivity of calcium phosphate makes it the perfect setting for the attachment and growth of bone cells [22, 23].

Materials made of calcium phosphate can be developed to be biodegradable in addition to being compatible with natural bone. For instance, tricalcium phosphate (TCP), a biodegradable variety of calcium phosphate, gradually dissolves over time to release calcium and phosphate ions, which are necessary for life [24].

In their work, Su et al. demonstrates that while there has been great progress made with CaP coated metallic implants in vitro and in vivo, there is still much work to be done before they can be used in clinical settings. In order to maximize the advantages of modern technology while minimizing its disadvantages, novel coating techniques should be investigated, especially when it comes to regulating the coating structures and degradation rate under mild coating circumstances. These are crucial factors in determining how well it functions biologically. The multilayer composite coating system is another emerging concept that will give biomedical implants multiple functions [25].

A brand-new bioactive endodontic sealer was created by Wang et al. with strong bond toughness to root canal dentine walls, nanoparticles of amorphous calcium phosphate (NACP) for remineralization, and powerful suppression of multispecies endodontic biofilms, lowering biofilm colony-forming units (CFU) by three log [26].

In their study, Balhaddad et al. discusses the development of caries, the role of pathogenic caries-related biofilm, the rise in the prevalence of CARS, and recent efforts to incorporate bioactive nanoparticles into rejuvenating polymer components as useful ways of managing and preventing caries-related bacteria. It was highlighted that the most developed and extensively studied interaction between calcium phosphate compounds and nanoparticle-based platforms in an effort to apply the promise of these strategies to dental clinical practise [27].

2.3.2 INTERACTION WITH LIVING TISSUES

A key component of calcium phosphate's bioactivity and biocompatibility is how it interacts with living tissues. Calcium phosphate substances create a dynamic link with the surrounding biological environment when they are introduced into the body [28]. The bone-forming cells called osteoblasts easily cling to the apatite-coated surface of calcium phosphate. This osteoconductivity makes it easier for osteoblasts to migrate and grow, which promotes the development of new bone tissue around the substance. The calcium phosphate scaffold gradually integrates into the developing bone as the bone tissue develops and expands, offering mechanical support and assisting in the repair of bone fractures or abnormalities [29]. Calcium phosphate can also be functionalized to transport bioactive chemicals and growth factors right to the target spot in addition to contributing to structure. By providing targeted therapeutic support, promoting cell activity, and altering the tissue milieu, this controlled drug delivery system improves tissue repair and regeneration [30].

For tissue regeneration, calcium phosphate's capacity to promote angiogenesis and vascularization is essential. An adequate supply of nutrients and oxygen is ensured through the establishment of new blood vessels within the designed tissue, promoting the growth of a functioning and viable tissue construct [31]. Additionally, calcium phosphate's bioactivity helps to modulate immune responses, minimise over-inflammation, and foster an environment that is conducive to tissue regeneration [31].

Biphasic and triphasic calcium phosphate fibres that resemble whiskers were used by Matinfar et al. to bolster porous frameworks made of chitosan (CS) and carboxymethyl cellulose (CMC). The results show that, despite the need for additional mechanical improvement, the created composite frameworks are feasible candidates for bone tissue engineering [32].

Biomineralized polyurethane (PU) foams were examined by Meskinfam et al. as a scaffold for regenerating bone tissue. When compared to untreated foams, biomineralization significantly increased the treated foams' mechanical qualities. The PU scaffold's cytocompatibility was also impacted by biomineralization, making it a better surface for cell adhesion and growth. Hence, the proposed scaffold can be regarded as suitable for bone tissue regeneration in light of the obtained results [33].

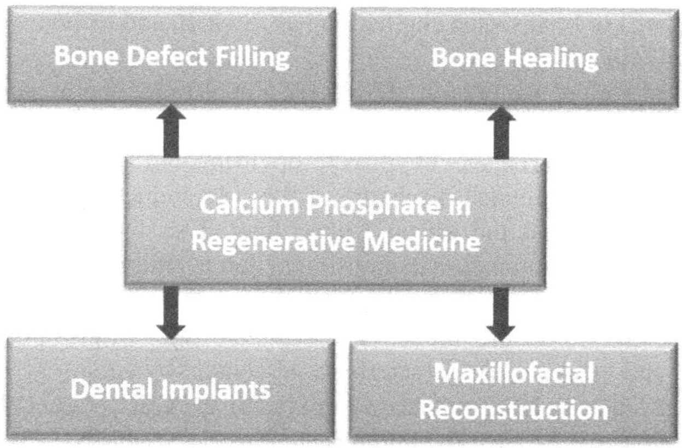

Figure 2.2 Application of calcium phosphate in regenerative medicines.

2.4 CLINICAL ADOPTION AND APPLICATIONS

The use of calcium phosphate in therapeutic settings has significantly advanced the science of regenerative medicine and enhanced patient outcomes across a range of medical disciplines. Calcium phosphate has been widely used in bone grafts, bone substitutes, and dental applications because it is a bioactive and biocompatible substance. It is the best option for fostering new bone formation and integration with the surrounding tissue in orthopaedic and dental procedures due to its capacity to enhance biomineralization and osteoconductivity [34]. Dental implants consisting of calcium phosphate-based materials have excelled at restoring both function and aesthetics in the mouth [35]. The various applications of calcium phosphate has been discussed herein and depicted in Figure 2.2.

2.4.1 BONE DEFECT FILLING

When bone defects arise as a result of fractures, trauma, or surgical procedures, the need for suitable materials to support bone regeneration and restoration is paramount [36]. The process of bone defect filling begins with the meticulous preparation of the defect site, ensuring a clean and stable environment for the implantation of calcium phosphate. The calcium phosphate substance is then gently inserted into the deficiency. It comes in granules, putty, or pre-formed shapes. By acting as an osteoconductive scaffold, the material's porous structure encourages the migration and proliferation of bone-forming cells like osteoblasts [37, 38]. Numerous benefits are associated with the successful use of calcium phosphate in bone defect filling, including a lower risk of adverse responses, a reduced inflammatory response, and a high level of biocompatibility with bone tissue [39]. It is a crucial tool in orthopaedic and reconstructive procedures due to its involvement in fostering bone regeneration and the restoration of bone integrity. Calcium phosphate's potential for filling bone defects is anticipated to significantly enhance patient outcomes and transform the area of bone tissue engineering as research and technological developments proceed [40].

In his investigation, Wang et al. developed a dual-functional bone-defect-filling substance with an arranged release system, which involves an explosive discharge of the powerful antibacterial agent hydroxypropyltrimethyl ammonium chloride chitosan (HACC) and a regulated discharge of the osteoinductive bone morphogenic protein (BMP2) to mend the affected bone flaw. The optimized HACC/BMP2-incorporated BioCaP combination demonstrated potent antibacterial activity and significantly increased osteoinduction when tested in vitro and in vivo [41].

In order to investigate the impact of micro-nano calcium phosphate (MNC) on the hydration and mechanical characteristics of cement by adding MNC to the Calcium phosphate and calcium sulphate cement (CPC and CSC), Cai et al. synthesized MNC with various Ca/P CSC. The findings demonstrate that MNC can influence cement crystal formation and can encourage the hydration reaction of CPC and CSC. The prepared concrete had the ability to be used in orthopaedic surgery to replace non-load-bearing bone deformities and were intended to resemble the new bone development in vivo [42]. The results are demonstrated in Figure 2.3.

Liu et al. discovered that BMP2-cop.BioCaP is an effective osteoinducer since it promoted bone formation and reduced the reactivity to alien bodies in critical-sized bone defects (CSBD) that had received a deproteinized bovine bone graft. Additionally, BMP2-cop.BioCaP has strong biocompatibility and degradation. Hence, it has a significant possibility as an osteoinducer to improve the curative benefits of the transplant components for the treatment of CSBD [43].

An injectable DNA-loaded nano-calcium phosphate paste that can serve as a bioactive bone replacement material was prepared by Schlickewei et al. After four

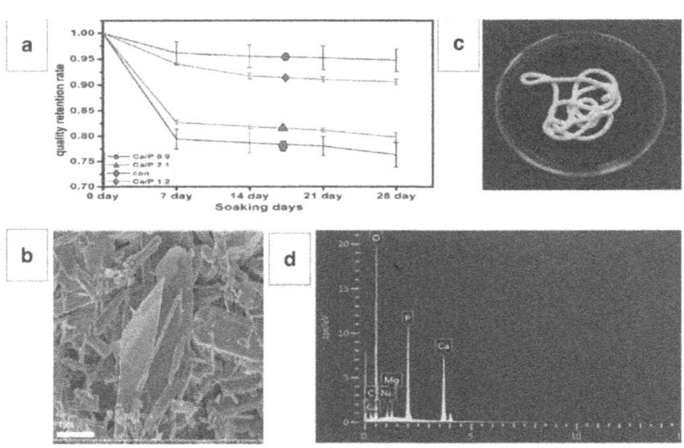

Figure 2.3 (a) The mass retaining rate of calcium sulphate cement with various MNC contents and (b) Fracture cross section of CSC samples as seen in a SEM picture [42]. (Reprinted from Cai *et al.* Copyrights Elsevier 2021.) (c) Images of DCP cement paste following injection and (d) BCP EDX spectra from lamb bone extraction [63]. (Reprinted from Tariq *et al.* Copyrights Elsevier 2019.)

weeks, the DNA-loaded bone paste caused the critical-size bone defect in the rabbit model to repair substantially more quickly. There was no discernible change in the new bone's condition. The paste caused an improved bone production as well as a more rapid and persistent bone repair. New bone emerged on the material's surface once it was thoroughly incorporated into the bone defect [44].

2.4.2 DENTAL IMPLANTS AND MAXILLOFACIAL RECONSTRUCTION

The utilization of calcium phosphate in dental implants and maxillofacial reconstruction exemplifies its versatility and significance in regenerative medicine [45].

By encouraging the creation of a bioactive apatite layer, calcium phosphate coatings for dental implants improve the osseointegration of the implant, resulting in higher implant durability and long-term success [46]. Additionally, bone grafts made of calcium phosphate are used to strengthen the jawbone, acting as a scaffold for the growth of new bone and aiding the integration of dental implants with the surrounding bone tissue. This encourages the efficient restoration of missing teeth as well as the aesthetics and optimal chewing function [47].

Calcium phosphate compounds are useful tools in maxillofacial reconstruction for mending and regenerating soft tissues and facial bones. Calcium phosphate scaffolds are used to fill bone deficiencies after trauma, congenital abnormalities, or tumor removal, promoting bone regeneration and integrating it with the surrounding tissues [48]. The particular facial architecture of each patient is taken into account while creating facial implants composed of calcium phosphate-based materials, allowing for the augmentation of facial contours and the restoration of facial symmetry [49]. Additionally, tissue engineering techniques use calcium phosphate scaffolds in more complicated maxillofacial reconstruction instances to encourage cell proliferation and organization, promoting the creation of useful tissues like bone, cartilage, or skin. This state-of-the-art calcium phosphate treatment has the potential to individually and precisely restore facial structure and function [50,51].

Ding et al. investigated 20 patients that underwent Maxillary Sinus Lift Surgery (MSLS) with a calcium phosphate graft filled with bone morphogenetic protein 2 (BMP2). In ten MSLS patients dental implants were implanted and in next ten MSLS patients dental implants were inserted three to six months later. Over a four to five year follow-up, the consequences were assessed based on medical and radiographic assessment. The results suggested that BMP2-loaded calcium phosphate would be an appropriate MSLS material, particularly for patients with low bone height [52].

In her work, Subira et al. demonstrated that with regard to their excellent percentage of survival, implants with modified calcium-phosphate surfaces could be the treatment option in clinical settings [53].

Arunjaroensuk et al. used biphasic calcium phosphate (BCP) with hydroxyapatite/tricalcium phosphate ratios of either 60/40 or 70/30 to examine the sustainability of the horizontal dimensions (facial bone thickness) of augmented bone. For shape enhancement concurrent with implant implantation, BCP bone grafts with HA/-TCP ratios of 60/40 and 70/30 demonstrated equivalent results. The 70/30 ratio, however, was remarkably superior in retaining face thickness and demonstrated more consistent horizontal dimensions of the augmented site [54].

2.4.3 ORTHOPEDIC APPLICATIONS FOR BONE HEALING

In orthopedic surgeries, such as fracture repair, spinal fusion, and joint replacements, promoting successful bone healing and integration is of utmost importance for restoring patients mobility and quality of life [55]. As a replacement for bone grafts, calcium phosphate is one of the main uses of the substance in orthopaedics [56]. Calcium phosphate materials, such as hydroxyapatite or tricalcium phosphate, can be used as bone grafts when patients have bone defects or inadequate bone volume to sustain the surgical intervention [57]. In order to facilitate cell adhesion and osteoconduction the process of directing bone-forming cells to migrate and deposit new bone matrix these materials offer a porous scaffold that mimics the structure of natural bone [58]. The patient's natural bone regenerates and integrates over time as the calcium phosphate scaffold is eventually replaced by new bone tissue [59].

Additionally, calcium phosphate materials are frequently utilized as bone graft extenders or replacements in spinal fusion operations, where two or more vertebrae are fused together to stabilize the spine and reduce pain [60].

Joint replacements have also used materials based on calcium phosphate. For example, calcium phosphate coatings are utilized to improve the osseointegration of the prosthetic components in total hip or knee arthroplasty. This increases the stability and durability of the implants, lowering the possibility of implant failure or loosening over time [61]. Further, calcium phosphate materials can be used to accelerate bone regeneration and support the natural healing process in situations of bone fractures that are difficult to repair, such as non-unions or delayed unions [62].

The manufacture of injectable bone cement using biphasic calcium phosphate (BCP) obtained from lamb femur bone by calcination is reported by Tariq et al. in his research. The findings show that bone cement made from BCP derived from femur lamb bone can be a possible bone replacement for bone regeneration and repair [63]. The results are demonstrated in Figure 2.3.

A new antibacterial framework made of chitosan-reinforced calcium phosphate cement that delivers doxycycline hyclate (CPCC + DOX) was created by Qiu et al. in his investigation. The new CPCC + DOX framework supported hPDLSC multiplication and osteogenic differentiation while displaying good mechanical capabilities and potent antibacterial activity. In dental, craniofacial, and orthopaedic applications, the CPCC + DOX + hPDLSCs architecture shows promise for promoting bone regeneration and preventing bone infections [64].

In his study, Mokhtari et al. created AZ31-calcium phosphate glass composites with a range of glass compositions (0–15 wt%). The findings showed that raising the glass particle quantity increased compressive strength and microhardness by 40% and 50%, respectively. Ultimately, it was discovered that the AZ31-calcium phosphate glass material has a significant potential for use as orthopaedic biodegradable implants due to its higher biocompatibility and adequate cell attachment in a material comprising 15 weight percent glass [65].

2.5 FUTURE PERSPECTIVE AND CONCLUSION

The long history of calcium phosphate in regenerative medicine demonstrates how important it is still today as a basic biomaterial. The ability of calcium phosphate to promote tissue repair and regeneration has been repeatedly established, from traditional treatments to contemporary biomedical uses. The potential for calcium phosphate in regenerative medicine are bright as we look to the future.

Technology advancements, like 3D printing and drug delivery systems, make it possible to develop calcium phosphate constructions that are highly personalized and patient-specific, maximizing their regeneration potential. Additionally, calcium phosphate in combination with other biomaterials and therapeutics will result in synergistic strategies that can more successfully treat complicated tissue injuries and disorders. The growing range of medical uses for calcium phosphate will continue to improve patient care by opening up new avenues for heart repair, nerve regeneration, and other processes. Calcium phosphate will continue to be a cornerstone of regenerative medicine as research and collaboration expand, revolutionizing tissue regeneration and restoration for countless people globally.

In conclusion, calcium phosphate's long history in regenerative medicine is evidence of both its worth and potential. With better results and a higher standard of living for patients, its bioactivity, biocompatibility, and osteoconductivity have revolutionized bone healing, dental implants, and maxillofacial reconstruction. The development of calcium phosphate in regenerative medicine is anticipated to continue as we move forward, leading the way for novel strategies and revolutionizing tissue healing and regeneration for future generations.

REFERENCES

1. S. Yamada, A. Behfar, and A. Terzic. Regenerative medicine clinical readiness. *Regenerative Medicine*, **16**(03):309–322, 2021.
2. R. M. Samsonraj, M. Raghunath, V. Nurcombe, J. H. Hui, A. J. van Wijnen, and S. M. Cool. Concise review: Multifaceted characterization of human mesenchymal stem cells for use in regenerative medicine. *Stem Cells Translational Medicine*, **6**(12):2173–2185, 2017.
3. D. Veeman, M. Swapna Sai, P. Sureshkumar, T. Jagadeesha, L. Natrayan, M. Ravichandran, and W. D. Mammo. Additive manufacturing of biopolymers for tissue engineering and regenerative medicine: An overview, potential applications, advancements, and trends. *International Journal of Polymer Science*, **2021**:1–20, 2021.
4. S. T. Boyce and A. L. Lalley. Tissue engineering of skin and regenerative medicine for wound care. *Burns & Trauma*, **6**:4, 2018.
5. G. Liu, J. Sun, M. Gong, F. Xing, S. Wu, and Z. Xiang. Urine-derived stem cells loaded onto a chitosan-optimized biphasic calcium-phosphate scaffold for repairing large segmental bone defects in rabbits. *Journal of Biomedical Materials Research Part B: Applied Biomaterials*, **109**(12):2014–2029, 2021.
6. J. Jeong, J. H. Kim, J. H. Shim, N. S. Hwang, and C. Y. Heo. Bioactive calcium phosphate materials and applications in bone regeneration. *Biomaterials Research*, **23**(1):1–11, 2019.

7. A. Salama. Recent progress in preparation and applications of chitosan/calcium phosphate composite materials. *International Journal of Biological Macromolecules*, **178**:240–252, 2021.
8. T. J. Levingstone, S. Herbaj, and N. J. Dunne. Calcium phosphate nanoparticles for therapeutic applications in bone regeneration. *Nanomaterials*, **9**(11):1570, 2019.
9. T. Brocke and J. Barr. The history of wound healing. *Surgical Clinics*, **100**(4):787–806, 2020.
10. E. Marin, F. Boschetto, and G. Pezzotti. Biomaterials and biocompatibility: An historical overview. *Journal of Biomedical Materials Research Part A*, **108**(8):1617–1633, 2020.
11. V. Singh. Medicinal plants and bone healing. *National Journal of Maxillofacial Surgery*, **8**(1):4, 2017.
12. S. A. A. Rizvi, G. P. Einstein, O. L. Tulp, F. Sainvil, and R. Branly. Introduction to traditional medicine and their role in prevention and treatment of emerging and re-emerging diseases. *Biomolecules*, **12**(10):1442, 2022.
13. J. Li and Y. Zhang. History of orthopaedics in China: A brief review. *International Orthopaedics*, **42**:713–717, 2018.
14. J. Lorkowski and M. Pokorski. Medical records: A historical narrative. *Biomedicines*, **10**(10):2594, 2022.
15. L. Grgurevic, M. Pecina, and S. Vukicevic. Marshall R. Urist and the discovery of bone morphogenetic proteins. *International Orthopaedics*, **41**:1065–1069, 2017.
16. S. K. Mishra and R. Chowdhary. Evolution of dental implants through the work of per-ingvar branemark: A systematic review. *Indian Journal of Dental Research*, **31**(6):930, 2020.
17. M. Montazerian and E. D. Zanotto. A guided walk through Larry Hench's monumental discoveries. *Journal of Materials Science*, **52**(15):8695–8732, 2017.
18. A. I. Caplan. Mesenchymal stem cells: Time to change the name! Stem Cells *Translational Medicine*, **6**(6):1445–1451, 2017.
19. I. Ielo, G. Calabrese, G. De Luca, and S. Conoci. Recent advances in hydroxyapatite-based biocomposites for bone tissue regeneration in orthopedics. *International Journal of Molecular Sciences*, **23**(17):9721, 2022.
20. S. Gautam, D. Bhatnagar, D. Bansal, H. Batra, and N. Goyal. Recent advancements in nanomaterials for biomedical implants. *Biomedical Engineering Advances*, **3**:100029, 2022.
21. L. Gritsch, G. Conoscenti, V. La Carrubba, P. Nooeaid, and A. R. Boccaccini. Polylactide-based materials science strategies to improve tissue-material interface without the use of growth factors or other biological molecules. *Materials Science and Engineering: C*, **94**:1083–1101, 2019.
22. S. K. Bhadada and S. D. Rao. Role of phosphate in biomineralization. *Calcified Tissue International*, **108**:32–40, 2021.
23. M. Bolean, A. M. S. Simão, M. B. Barioni, B. Z. Favarin, H. G. Sebinelli, E. A. Veschi, T. A. B. Janku, M. Bottini, M. F. Hoylaerts, R. Itri, J. L. Millán and P. Ciancaglini. Biophysical aspects of biomineralization. *Biophysical Reviews*, **9**:747–760, 2017.
24. K. Kúsnierczyk and M. Basista. Recent advances in research on magnesium alloys and magnesium-calcium phosphate composites as biodegradable implant materials. *Journal of Biomaterials Applications*, **31**(6):878–900, 2017.
25. Y. Su, I. Cockerill, Y. Zheng, L. Tang, Y.-X. Qin, and D. Zhu. Biofunctionalization of metallic implants by calcium phosphate coatings. *Bioactive Materials*, **4**:196–206, 2019.

26. L. Wang, X. Xie, C. Li, H. Liu, K. Zhang, Y. Zhou, X. Chang, and H. H. K. Xu. Novel bioactive root canal sealer to inhibit endodontic multispecies biofilms with remineralizing calcium phosphate ions. *Journal of Dentistry*, **60**:25–35, 2017.
27. A. A. Balhaddad, A. A. Kansara, D. Hidan, M. D. Weir, H. H. K. Xu, and M. A. S. Melo. Toward dental caries: Exploring nanoparticle-based platforms and calcium phosphate compounds for dental restorative materials. *Bioactive Materials*, **4**:43–55, 2019.
28. S. E. Kim and K. Park. Recent advances of biphasic calcium phosphate bioceramics for bone tissue regeneration. In: Chun, H., Reis, R., Motta, A., Khang, G. (eds). *Biomimicked Biomaterials: Advances in Experimental Medicine and Biology*, **1250**. Springer: Singapore. 2020.
29. V. Sharma, Al. Srinivasan, F. Nikolajeff, and S. Kumar. Biomineralization process in hard tissues: The interaction complexity within protein and inorganic counterparts. *Acta Biomaterialia*, **120**:20–37, 2021.
30. V. Sokolova and M. Epple. Biological and medical applications of calcium phosphate nanoparticles. *Chemistry–A European Journal*, **27**(27):7471–7488, 2021.
31. Y. Lin, S. Huang, R. Zou, X. Gao, J. Ruan, M. D. Weir, M. A. Reynolds, W. Qin, X. Chang, H. Fu, and H. H. K. Xu. Calcium phosphate cement scaffold with stem cell co-culture and prevascularization for dental and craniofacial bone tissue engineering. *Dental Materials*, **35**(7):1031–1041, 2019.
32. M. Matinfar, A. S. Mesgar, and Z. Mohammadi. Evaluation of physicochemical, mechanical and biological properties of chitosan/carboxymethyl cellulose reinforced with multiphasic calcium phosphate whisker-like fibers for bone tissue engineering. *Materials Science and Engineering: C*, **100**:341–353, 2019.
33. M. Meskinfam, S. Bertoldi, N. Albanese, A. Cerri, M. C. Tanzi, R. Imani, N. Baheiraei, M. Farokhi, and S. Fare. Polyurethane foam/nano hydroxyapatite composite as a suitable scaffold for bone tissue regeneration. *Materials Science and Engineering: C*, **82**:130–140, 2018.
34. H. H. K. Xu, P. Wang, L. Wang, C. Bao, Q. Chen, M. D. Weir, L. C. Chow, L. Zhao, X. Zhou, and M. A. Reynolds. Calcium phosphate cements for bone engineering and their biological properties. *Bone Research*, **5**(1):1–19, 2017.
35. H. R. Fernandes, A. Gaddam, A. Rebelo, D. Brazete, G. E. Stan, and J. M. F. Ferreira. Bioactive glasses and glass-ceramics for healthcare applications in bone regeneration and tissue engineering. *Materials*, **11**(12):2530, 2018.
36. J. R. Perez, D. Kouroupis, D. J. Li, T. M. Best, L. Kaplan, and D. Correa. Tissue engineering and cell-based therapies for fractures and bone defects. *Frontiers in Bioengineering and Biotechnology*, **6**:105, 2018.
37. L. He, J. Yin, and X. Gao. Additive manufacturing of bioactive glass and its polymer composites as bone tissue engineering scaffolds: A review. *Bioengineering*, **10**(6):672, 2023.
38. H.-S. Sohn and J.-K. Oh. Review of bone graft and bone substitutes with an emphasis on fracture surgeries. *Biomaterials Research*, **23**(1):1–7, 2019.
39. G. Fernandez de Grado, L. Keller, Y. Idoux-Gillet, Q. Wagner, A.-M. Musset, N. Benkirane-Jessel, F. Bornert, and D. Offner. Bone substitutes: A review of their characteristics, clinical use, and perspectives for large bone defects management. *Journal of Tissue Engineering*, **9**:2041731418776819, 2018.
40. G. L. Koons, M. Diba, and A. G. Mikos. Materials design for bone-tissue engineering. *Nature Reviews Materials*, **5**(8):584–603, 2020.

41. D. Wang, Y. Liu, Y. Liu, L. Yan, S. A. J. Zaat, D. Wismeijer, J. L. Pathak, and G. Wu. A dual functional bone-defect-filling material with sequential antibacterial and osteoinductive properties for infected bone defect repair. *Journal of Biomedical Materials Research Part A*, **107**(10):2360–2370, 2019.
42. Z. Cai, Z. Wu, Y. Wan, T. Yu, and C. Zhou. Manipulation of the degradation behavior of calcium phosphate and calcium sulfate bone cement system by the addition of micro-nano calcium phosphate. *Ceramics International*, **47**(20):29213–29224, 2021.
43. T. Liu, Y. Zheng, G. Wu, D. Wismeijer, J. L. Pathak, and Y. Liu. BMP2-coprecipitated calcium phosphate granules enhance osteoinductivity of deproteinized bovine bone, and bone formation during critical-sized bone defect healing. *Scientific Reports*, **7**(1):41800, 2017.
44. C. Schlickewei, T. O. Klatte, Y. Wildermuth, G. Laaff, J. M. Rueger, J. Ruesing, S. Chernousova, W. Lehmann, and M. Epple. A bioactive nano-calcium phosphate paste for in-situ transfection of BMP-7 and VEGF-A in a rabbit critical-size bone defect: Results of an in vivo study. *Journal of Materials Science: Materials in Medicine*, **30**:1–12, 2019.
45. J. H. Oh. Recent advances in the reconstruction of cranio-maxillofacial defects using computer-aided design/computer-aided manufacturing. *Maxillofacial Plastic and Reconstructive Surgery*, **40**(1):2, 2018.
46. F. H. Schünemann, M. E. Galárraga-Vinueza, R. Magini, M. Fredel, F. Silva, J. C. M. Souza, Y. Zhang, and B. Henriques. Zirconia surface modifications for implant dentistry. *Materials Science and Engineering: C*, **98**:1294–1305, 2019.
47. S. Titsinides, G. Agrogiannis, and T. Karatzas. Bone grafting materials in dentoalveolar reconstruction: A comprehensive review. *Japanese Dental Science Review*, **55**(1):26–32, 2019.
48. N. T. Moussa and H. Dym. Maxillofacial bone grafting materials. *Dental Clinics*, **64**(2):473–490, 2020.
49. A. A. Raheem, P. Hameed, R. Whenish, R. S. Elsen, A. K. Jaiswal, K. G. Prashanth, and G. Manivasagam. A review on development of bio-inspired implants using 3D printing. *Biomimetics*, **6**(4):65, 2021.
50. G. Ceccarelli, R. Presta, L. Benedetti, M. G. C. De Angelis, S. M. Lupi, R. Rodriguez y Baena, et al. Emerging perspectives in scaffold for tissue engineering in oral surgery. *Stem Cells International*, Article ID 4585401, **2017**, 2017.
51. M. Alonzo, F. A. Primo, S. A. Kumar, J. A. Mudloff, E. Dominguez, G. Fregoso, N. Ortiz, W. M. Weiss, and B. Joddar. Bone tissue engineering techniques, advances, and scaffolds for treatment of bone defects. *Current Opinion in Biomedical Engineering*, **17**:100248, 2021.
52. Y. Ding and X. Wang. Long-term effects of bone morphogenetic protein-2–loaded calcium phosphate on maxillary sinus lift surgery for delayed and simultaneous dental implantation. *Journal of Craniofacial Surgery*, **29**(1):e58–e61, 2018.
53. C. Subirà-Pifarré, C. Masuet-Aumatell, C. R. Alonso, R. M. Madrid, and C. Galletti. Assessment of dental implants with modified calcium-phosphate surface in a multicenter, prospective, non-interventional study: Results up to 50 months of follow-up. *Journal of Functional Biomaterials*, **10**(1):5, 2019.
54. S. Arunjaroensuk, P. Thunyakitpisal, K. Nampuksa, N. Monmaturapoj, N. Mattheos, and A. Pimkhaokham. Stability of guided bone regeneration with two ratios of biphasic calcium phosphate at implant sites in the esthetic zone: A randomized controlled clinical trial. *Clinical Oral Implants Research*, **34**(8):850–862, 2023.

55. K. Pawelec and J. A. Planell. Bone Repair Biomaterials: Regeneration and Clinical Applications. **1**, chapter 11, second edition, 2018.
56. M. W. Archunan and S. Petronis. Bone grafts in trauma and orthopaedics. *Cureus*, **13**(9):e17705, 2021.
57. M. Bohner, B. Le Gars Santoni, and N. Döbelin. β-tricalcium phosphate for bone substitution: Synthesis and properties. *Acta Biomaterialia*, **113**:23–41, 2020.
58. D. A. Florea, C. Chircov, and A. M. Grumezescu. Hydroxyapatite particlesdirecting the cellular activity in bone regeneration processes: An up-to-date review. *Applied Sciences*, **10**(10):3483, 2020.
59. F. Pupilli, A. Ruffini, M. Dapporto, M. Tavoni, A. Tampieri, and S. Sprio. Design strategies and biomimetic approaches for calcium phosphate scaffolds in bone tissue regeneration. *Biomimetics*, **7**(3):112, 2022.
60. M. A. Plantz, E. B. Gerlach, and W. K. Hsu. Synthetic bone graft materials in spine fusion: Current evidence and future trends. *International Journal of Spine Surgery*, **15**(s1):104–112, 2021.
61. A.-M. Yousefi. A review of calcium phosphate cements and acrylic bone cements as injectable materials for bone repair and implant fixation. *Journal of Applied Biomaterials & Functional Materials*, **17**(4):2280800019872594, 2019.
62. I. Lodoso-Torrecilla, J. J. J. P. van den Beucken, and J. A. Jansen. Calcium phosphate cements: Optimization toward biodegradability. *Acta Biomaterialia*, **119**:1–12, 2021.
63. U. Tariq, R. Hussain, K. Tufail, Z. Haider, R. Tariq, and J. Ali. Injectable dicalcium phosphate bone cement prepared from biphasic calcium phosphate extracted from lamb bone. *Materials Science and Engineering: C*, **103**:109863, 2019.
64. G. Qiu, M. Huang, J. Liu, P. Wang, A. Schneider, K. Ren, T. W. Oates, M. D. Weir, H. H. K. Xu, and L. Zhao. Antibacterial calcium phosphate cement with human periodontal ligament stem cell-microbeads to enhance bone regeneration and combat infection. *Journal of Tissue Engineering and Regenerative Medicine*, **15**(3):232–243, 2021.
65. S. Mokhtari, B. E. Yekta, V. Marghussian, and P. T. Ahmadi. Synthesis and characterization of biodegradable AZ31/calcium phosphate glass composites for orthopedic applications. *Advanced Composites and Hybrid Materials*, **3**:390–401, 2020.

3 Clinical Applications of Calcium Phosphates in Orthopaedics

Dhruv Bhatnagar and Sanjeev Gautam
Advanced Functional Materials Laboratory, Dr. S.S. Bhatnagar University Institute of Chemical Engineering and Technology, Panjab University, Chandigarh, India

3.1 INTRODUCTION

Orthopedic conditions and injuries pose significant challenges in healthcare, requiring effective interventions to restore bone function and promote healing [1]. Calcium phosphates have emerged as a versatile class of biomaterials with numerous clinical applications in the field of orthopedics. These materials exhibit unique properties that make them highly valuable for a range of orthopedic procedures, including bone graft substitutes, tissue engineering scaffolds, dental implants, biocompatible coatings, drug delivery systems, and calcium phosphate cements for bone fillers [2, 3]. The structural and compositional similarity between calcium phosphates and the mineral components of bone, particularly hydroxyapatite (HA), has driven their extensive use in orthopedics. HA, the primary inorganic component of bone, provides excellent biocompatibility and osteoconductivity, enabling the integration of calcium phosphates with host bone tissue [4]. This integration facilitates bone regeneration and remodeling, making calcium phosphates an attractive choice for orthopedic applications [5].

In this comprehensive book chapter, the clinical applications of calcium phosphates in orthopedics is explored, shedding light on their diverse utility and their impact on patient outcomes. Calcium phosphate compounds encompass a variety of materials, including hydroxyapatite (HA), tricalcium phosphate (TCP), and biphasic calcium phosphate (BCP). HA is the most commonly used calcium phosphate material in orthopedics due to its similarities to the mineral phase of bone [6, 7]. HA possesses a hexagonal crystal structure and a stoichiometric composition of $Ca_{10}(PO_4)_6(OH)_2$. TCP, on the other hand, has a more soluble nature and can be found in various forms, such as β- and α-TCP, with different crystal structures and dissolution rates [8, 9]. BCP consists of a mixture of HA and TCP, providing

DOI: 10.1201/9781003360605-3

a balance between their properties. The crystal structure and composition of calcium phosphates play a crucial role in determining their properties and behavior in orthopedic applications [10]. HA's crystal structure provides stability, while the presence of hydroxyl groups contributes to its bioactivity [11]. The ratio of calcium to phosphate ions affects the solubility and dissolution behavior of calcium phosphates, influencing their osteoconductivity and ability to release calcium and phosphate ions, which are essential for bone regeneration [12].

Bone grafting is a common procedure to fill bone defects and promote bone healing. Calcium phosphate materials, such as HA and TCP, have demonstrated excellent biocompatibility and osteoconductivity, enabling the gradual resorption and replacement by the host bone [13]. These materials can be used alone or in combination with other substances, such as autografts or growth factors, to enhance bone healing outcomes. Another important application is the use of calcium phosphates as scaffolds in tissue engineering approaches for orthopedic regeneration [14]. These scaffolds provide a three-dimensional structure that supports cell attachment, proliferation, and differentiation, mimicking the natural extracellular matrix. By seeding the scaffold with bone-forming cells, such as mesenchymal stem cells (MSCs), and providing appropriate growth factors, calcium phosphate scaffolds can facilitate the regeneration of bone tissue [15, 16]. The interconnected porosity of these scaffolds allows for nutrient and oxygen diffusion, promoting cell viability and tissue ingrowth. In the field of dental implantology, calcium phosphates have found valuable applications. Dental implants require successful osseointegration, where the implant fuses with the surrounding bone tissue. Calcium phosphate coatings on dental implants enhance osseointegration by promoting direct bone apposition onto the implant surface [17]. These coatings improve the implant's stability and long-term clinical performance, leading to successful and durable dental implant restorations [18]. Calcium phosphates offer a unique advantage as drug delivery systems in orthopedics. By incorporating therapeutic agents, such as antibiotics or growth factors, into the calcium phosphate matrix, localized and controlled drug release can be achieved [19]. This targeted delivery allows for the precise administration of therapeutic agents to specific areas requiring intervention, such as bone defects or infected sites associated with orthopedic implants. The slow and sustained release of drugs from the calcium phosphate matrix enhances their therapeutic efficacy while minimizing systemic side effects [20]. Studies on calcium phosphate coatings have shown improved implant fixation and reduced rates of implant-related complications [21]. Furthermore, clinical investigations on calcium phosphate cements have highlighted their utility in various orthopedic procedures, including spine surgery and joint arthroplasty.

As research and technological advancements continue, the future of calcium phosphates in orthopedics looks promising. The development of composite materials, improved drug delivery systems, and the integration of advanced technologies, such as additive manufacturing or tissue engineering approaches, hold the potential for further enhancing bone regeneration and patient outcomes [22]. In conclusion, calcium phosphates offer a broad range of clinical applications in orthopedics, addressing the challenges associated with bone defects, fractures, and implant-related complications. Their unique properties, including biocompatibility, osteoconductivity, and the ability to mimic bone mineral components, position them as valuable biomaterials in orthopedic interventions. As our understanding of calcium phosphates expands and new technologies emerge, their role in orthopedics is likely to continue growing, offering improved treatments and outcomes for patients with orthopedic conditions.

3.2 STRUCTURE AND TYPES OF CALCIUM PHOSPHATE

Calcium phosphate compounds are characterized by their crystal structure, composition, and various types. These compounds consist of calcium ions (Ca^{2+}) and phosphate ions ($PO_4{}^{3-}$). One prominent type is hydroxyapatite(HAp), which is the main mineral component of bone and teeth. It has a hexagonal crystal structure and the chemical formula $Ca_{10}(PO_4)_6(OH)_2$ [23]. Another type is dicalcium phosphate dihydrate (DCPD), also known as brushite, which has a monoclinic crystal structure and the chemical formula $CaHPO_4{\cdot}2H_2O$. Octacalcium phosphate (OCP) is another calcium phosphate compound with a complex layered crystal structure and the formula $Ca_8(HPO_4)_2(PO_4)_4{\cdot}5H_2O$ [24]. Monetite, or calcium phosphate monobasic, adopts a monoclinic crystal structure and has the formula $CaHPO_4$. Additionally, amorphous calcium phosphate (ACP) lacks a well-defined crystal structure and exists as a non-crystalline or semi-crystalline material [25]. The diverse crystal structures and compositions of calcium phosphate compounds contribute to their wide range of applications in fields such as medicine, dentistry, and biomaterials.

3.2.1 CRYSTAL STRUCTURE AND COMPOSITION OF CALCIUM PHOSPHATE

The crystal structure of calcium phosphate compounds can vary depending on the specific compound. One of the most common calcium phosphate structures is hydroxyapatite (HAp), which has a hexagonal crystal structure. In HAp, calcium ions (Ca^{2+}) and phosphate ions ($PO_4{}^{3-}$) are arranged in a repeating pattern, with hydroxyl groups (OH^-) occupying interstitial sites [26]. Another calcium phosphate compound, dicalcium phosphate dihydrate (DCPD) or brushite, exhibits a monoclinic crystal structure. DCPD consists of calcium ions, phosphate ions, and water molecules arranged in layers within the crystal structure [27]. Octacalcium phosphate (OCP) has a more complex crystal structure, consisting of alternating layers of calcium ions and phosphate ions stacked in a specific arrangement. Monetite, another calcium phosphate compound, shares a similar monoclinic crystal structure with brushite. It contains calcium ions and phosphate ions, but their arrangement differs from that of DCPD [28]. It's important to note that amorphous calcium phosphate (ACP) lacks a well-defined crystal structure and is instead a disordered or semicrystalline material. These various crystal structures contribute to the unique properties and applications of calcium phosphate compounds in fields such as biomedicine, dentistry, and materials science.

Wang et al. [29] synthesized strontium (Sr) doped biphasic calcium phosphate (BCP) with different Sr concentrations of 1, 5, and 15 mol% using chemical precipitation and a high-temperature calcination method. The XRD data and rietveld refinement results shows the decrease in HAp percentage, distorted HAp structure, and less stability of HAp structure. Although, in 15 mol% Sr doped the concentration of HAp rises which results in increase in lattice constants and volume of the composite. The XPS result reveals that Sr is not only on the surface of sample but also it is present in crystalline structure of HAp. He et al. [30] synthesized Sr doped hydroxyapatite (HAp) powders using chemical precipitation technique. The phase transformation analysis and quantitative analysis was done using X-ray diffraction and rietveld analysis. The lattice parameters increased and also the binding energy of the Ca was enhanced by the doping of Sr in the samples. The results are very promising and Sr incorporation makes the calcium phosphate an effective material for bone repair.

The various types of calcium phosphate compounds exhibit distinct structures and play crucial roles in numerous fields, owing to their biocompatibility and functional properties.

3.2.2 DIFFERENT FORMS OF CALCIUM PHOSPHATE

Calcium phosphate is found in various forms, each with distinct characteristics and applications. Hydroxyapatite (HA) is the most common and stable form, serving as the primary mineral component of bones and teeth. It is biocompatible and widely used in biomedical applications [31]. Dicalcium phosphate (DCP) encompasses different hydrated forms like monetite and brushite, finding applications in pharmaceuticals, food additives, and dental products. Octacalcium phosphate (OCP) acts as an intermediate phase in bone mineralization and is involved in early-stage bone repair [32]. Amorphous calcium phosphate (ACP) lacks a defined crystal structure and offers enhanced solubility and bioactivity, making it useful in remineralization treatments and coatings [33]. Beta-tricalcium phosphate (β-TCP) is a bioresorbable material commonly employed in bone grafting due to its osteoconductive properties [34]. Alpha-tricalcium phosphate (α-TCP), with higher crystallinity and slower resorption rate, is used in dental materials and ceramics.

Lotsari et al. [35] observed the transformation of spherical calcium phosphate particles to bone-like apatite structure. The change take place in the presence of humidity as crystallization proceeds due to migration of nanometer clusters. The HR-TEM revealed that step-growth mechanism lead to transformation and crystal growth. It was concluded that step-growth mechanism can explain the irregularity in bone apatite structure that can describe the stages in bone mineralization.

The diverse forms of calcium phosphate can play an important role in different biomedical applications and as explained above can be transformed from one form to another using different techniques.

3.3 APPLICATION OF CALCIUM PHOSPHATE IN ORTHOPEDICS

Calcium phosphate has a wide range of applications in orthopedics, making it a valuable material in the field. It has several biomedical applications as shown in

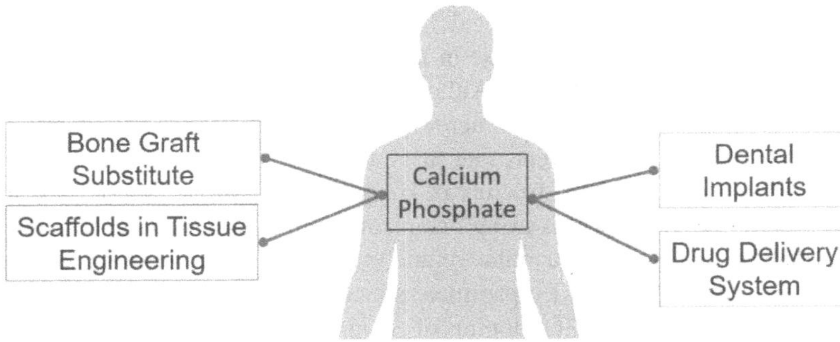

Figure 3.1 Diagram showing different applications of calcium phosphate.

Figure 3.1. One key application is in bone grafting, where calcium phosphate-based materials such as hydroxyapatite (HA) and tricalcium phosphate (TCP) serve as bone graft substitutes [36]. These materials provide a scaffold that promotes new bone growth and integration with existing bone, aiding in the healing of fractures or bone defects. Additionally, calcium phosphate cements are utilized as bone void fillers, providing immediate structural support and gradually being replaced by new bone over time [37]. Calcium phosphate coatings are applied to orthopedic implants to enhance osseointegration, improving the bond between the implant and surrounding bone. Moreover, calcium phosphate scaffolds act as osteoconductive frameworks, stimulating bone regeneration in large defects [38]. The versatility of calcium phosphate also extends to drug delivery systems, with calcium phosphate nanoparticles or microparticles used as carriers for targeted release of therapeutic agents at the site of bone injury or infection [39]. The use of calcium phosphate in orthopedics benefits patients by facilitating bone healing, promoting implant stability, and improving overall outcomes in various orthopedic procedures.

3.3.1 BONE GRAFT SUBSTITUTES

Bone graft substitutes are materials used in orthopedic and dental surgeries to replace deficient bone tissue. These substitutes serve as alternatives to traditional autografts or allografts, offering various advantages such as reduced donor site morbidity, unlimited availability, and elimination of disease transmission risks [41]. Calcium phosphate plays a significant role in bone graft substitutes, contributing to their effectiveness in bone regeneration and repair. Calcium phosphate-based materials, such as hydroxyapatite (HA) and tricalcium phosphate (TCP), are commonly used in bone graft substitutes due to their biocompatibility and resemblance to natural bone mineral [42, 43]. These materials provide a scaffold for new bone formation and facilitate the attachment, migration, and proliferation of bone cells. The porous structure of calcium phosphate scaffolds allows for the infiltration of cells and the exchange of nutrients, promoting the formation of new tissue [44].

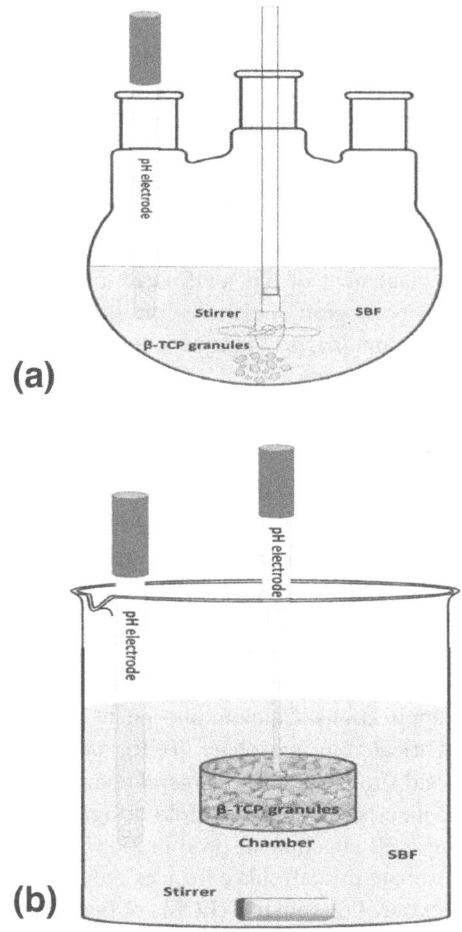

Figure 3.2 Experimental setup (a) Unconfined and (b) confined to test to examine the chemical alterations inside the calcium phosphate granules using SBF solution [40]. (Reprinted from Maazouz *et al.* Copyrights Elsevier 2020.)

Beslega et al. [45] fabricated Mg and Sr doped Bi-phasic calcium phosphate using hydrothermal synthesis technique for application as bone-graft substitutes. The in-vitro performance of the prepared samples were investigated using various physical and chemical techniques. The results revealed that all the samples show good biocompatibility and similar in-vitro performance. Mg and Sr were found to be predominantly incorporated in the β-TCP lattice and also β-TCP shows higher dissolution rate useful for application as bone graft substitute. Maazouz et al. [40] investigated the chemical alterations taking place inside the pores of β-Tricalcium phosphate granules incubated in a simulated body fluid using a quick and quantitative approach. The experimental setup used in the researchs has been presented in the Figure 3.2. The changes in calcium, and phosphate concentration, and also the change in pH was observed inside the granules. It was concluded that the model may be beneficial to predict the osteoinductive potential of calcium phosphate granules. The processing factors that enhanced the kinetics and amplitude of the local chemical changes are also thought to favor calcium phosphate osteoinduction which is the interesting observation.

Moreover, calcium phosphate-based graft substitutes can be engineered to have specific compositions and degradation rates, tailoring their properties to match the needs of the defect being treated. The biodegradability of calcium phosphate allows for the gradual replacement of the scaffold by new bone over time. The use of calcium phosphate in bone graft substitutes offers a valuable solution for bone defects, fractures, and non-unions, providing structural support and promoting successful bone healing and integration.

3.3.2 SCAFFOLDS IN TISSUE ENGINEERING

Scaffolds play a crucial role in tissue engineering by providing a framework for cell attachment, proliferation, and differentiation, ultimately promoting the regeneration of functional tissues. These three-dimensional structures mimic the extracellular matrix (ECM) and create a microenvironment that supports cellular activities [48]. Scaffolds are designed with specific pore sizes, interconnected networks, and material compositions to facilitate nutrient and oxygen diffusion, waste removal, and cell-cell communication [49]. Calcium phosphate plays a crucial role in scaffolds for tissue engineering applications. Calcium phosphate-based materials, such as hydroxyapatite (HA) and tricalcium phosphate (TCP), are commonly utilized due to their biocompatibility and similarity to the mineral component of natural bone [50]. These materials can be incorporated into scaffold designs to provide a bioactive environment that promotes cell attachment, proliferation, and differentiation. The inclusion of calcium phosphate in scaffolds enhances the scaffold's osteoconductivity and mimics the native extracellular matrix (ECM) of bone tissue [51].

Touri et al. [46] fabricated 60% hydroxyapatite (HA) and 40% β-tricalcium phosphate (β-TCP) scaffolds using a direct-write assembly technique. Then, the scaffolds were coated with calcium peroxide (CPO) and used for production of oxygen at implanted sites. The results revealed that 3% CPO coated samples has a strong potential for enhancing bone ingrowth by increasing osteoblast cells' viability and proliferation. The results are very promising and oxygen diffusion property as shown in Figure 3.3 can be helpful in designing further scaffolds in tissue engineering.

Additionally, calcium phosphate scaffolds can be tailored to have specific degradation rates, allowing for the gradual release of calcium and phosphate ions, which are essential for stimulating bone cell activity and facilitating tissue regeneration. The presence of calcium phosphate in scaffolds used in tissue engineering offers a biomimetic and supportive framework for the growth and development of new tissue, making it a valuable component in promoting successful tissue regeneration and repair.

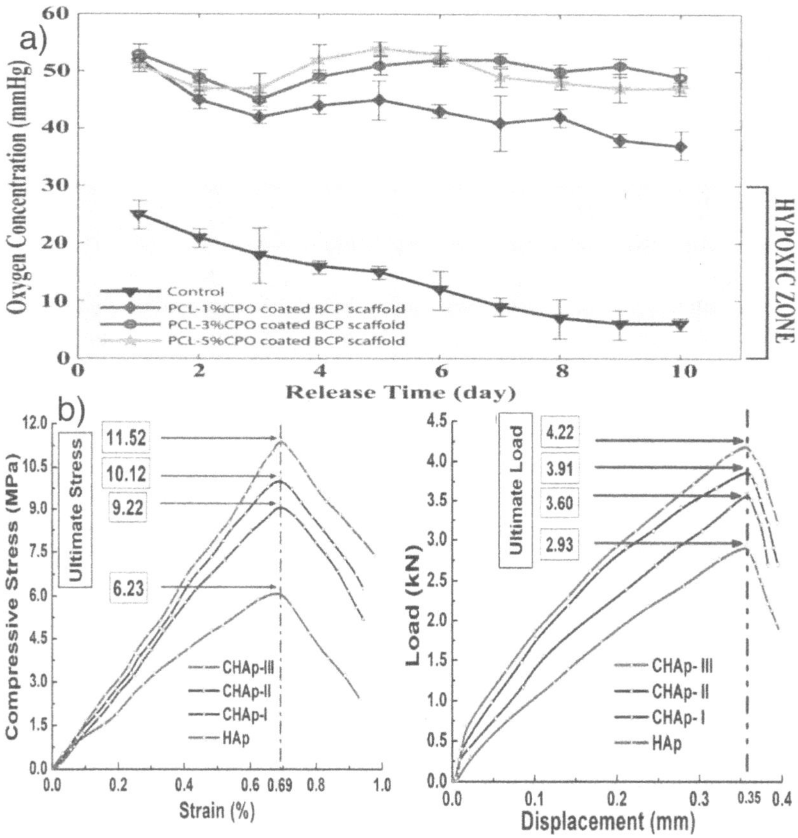

Figure 3.3 (a) Oxygen production behavior of coated scaffolds with varying calcium peroxide concentrations [46]. (Reprinted from Touri *et al.* Copyrights Elsevier 2018.) (b) Variation of compressive strength and fracture toughness with different carbonate content [47]. (Reprinted from Bhatnagar *et al.* Copyrights Elsevier 2023).

3.3.3 DENTAL IMPLANTS

Dental implants are prosthetic devices used to replace missing teeth and restore oral function and aesthetics. They consist of three main components: the implant fixture, abutment, and dental crown [54]. The implant fixture, typically made of biocompatible titanium, is surgically placed into the jawbone, and serves as an artificial tooth root. Over time, the implant integrates with the bone through a process called osseointegration, providing a stable foundation for the replacement tooth [55]. The abutment connects the implant fixture to the dental crown and acts as a connector. The dental crown, custom-made to match the shape, size, and color of the surrounding teeth, is attached to the abutment, creating a natural-looking and functional replacement tooth [56]. Calcium phosphate has significant applications in dental implants, contributing to their success in restorative dentistry. Calcium phosphate coatings are often applied to dental implant surfaces to enhance osseointegration, the process by which the implant fuses with the surrounding bone [57]. These coatings promote better bone cell attachment and integration, leading to improved stability and long-term success of the implant. The use of calcium phosphate in dental implant coatings provides a bioactive surface that encourages bone formation and remodeling [58]. Additionally, calcium phosphate materials, such as hydroxyapatite (HA) or tricalcium phosphate (TCP), can be incorporated into implant materials to enhance their bioactivity and stimulate bone regeneration.

Bhatnagar et al. [47] investigated the structural and mechanical properties of carbonated hydroxyapatite synthesized using hydrothermal synthesis technique. The samples were characterized by Rietveld analysis and mechanical testing. The results revealed that the substitution of carbonate in HAp samples significantly enhanced the fracture toughness and compressive strength of the samples as shown in Figure 3.3. It was concluded that further studies can also be done to study the effect of carbonate substitution on hydroxyapatite for application as biomedical implant material. Schickert et al. [52] assessed the fiber-reinforced calcium phosphate cements' ability to stabilize dental implants both in vitro and in vivo, using a variety of mechanical and biological test techniques. The fiber-reinforced samples shows better implant stability as shown by histological images mentioned in Figure 3.4 and also the superior osteocompatibility property in calcium phosphate samples reinforced by fiber. It was concluded that fiber-reinforced samples can stabilize the dental implants during osseointegration.

Dental implants offer several advantages, including improved chewing and speaking ability, enhanced oral health, preservation of jawbone structure, and enhanced aesthetics. The application of calcium phosphate in dental implants plays a

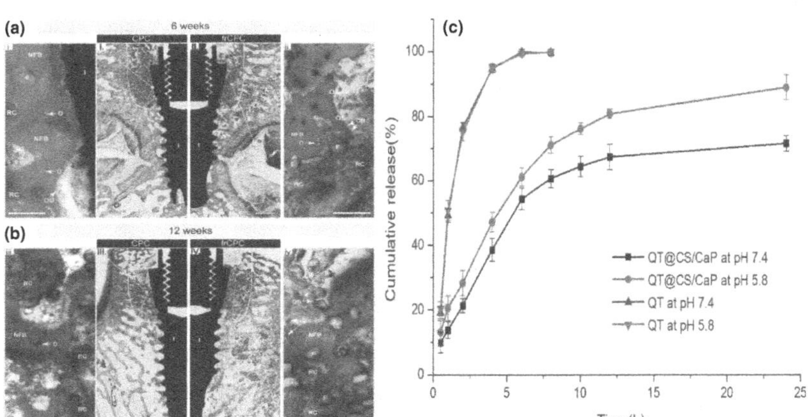

Figure 3.4 Histological images after (a) 6 weeks of implantation. (b) 12 weeks of implantation [52]. (Reprinted from Schickert *et al.* Copyrights Elsevier 2020.), (c) Drug release behavior prepared samples in pH 5.8 and 7.4 [53]. (Reprinted from Luo *et al.* Copyrights Elsevier 2020.)

vital role in optimizing their biocompatibility, osseointegration, and long-term functionality in dental restorations.

3.3.4 DRUG DELIVERY SYSTEMS

Drug delivery systems are designed to efficiently deliver therapeutic agents to specific target sites in the body, providing controlled and sustained release of medications. These systems aim to optimize drug efficacy while minimizing side effects and improving patient compliance [59]. Drug delivery systems can take various forms, including implants, patches, nanoparticles, liposomes, microspheres, and hydrogels [60]. They can be designed to release drugs in response to specific triggers, such as pH, temperature, or enzymes, or to provide sustained release over an extended period. Calcium phosphate has significant applications in drug delivery systems, contributing to their effectiveness in targeted and controlled drug release [61]. Calcium phosphate nanoparticles or microparticles are commonly used as carriers for drug delivery due to their biocompatibility, biodegradability, and tunable properties [62]. These particles can encapsulate a variety of therapeutic agents, such as small molecules, proteins, peptides, or nucleic acids, protecting them from degradation and facilitating their controlled release at the desired site. Calcium phosphate particles can be engineered to have specific sizes, surface charges, and degradation rates, allowing for customization of drug release kinetics [63, 64]. Additionally, the surface of calcium phosphate particles can be modified to improve stability, enhance targeting capabilities, or enable triggered release in response to specific stimuli.

Luo et al. [53] fabricated a drug release system using chitosan and calcium phosphate microparticle. The SEM and TEM microscopy was used to study morphology and in-vitro studies is done to study release kinetics and pH properties. The microscopy revealed the flower-like structure with 5–7 μm diameter. the in-vitro studies suggested no cytotoxic behavior and also a well-sustained release mechanism of prepared samples as shown in Figure 3.4. He et al. [65] synthesized a nanodrug delivery system in which calcium phosphate precursor is doped into silica matrix one-step growth technique. The drug loading release mechanism is being tested. The mesoporous silica-calcium phosphate nano carrier exhibited a high doxorubicin (DOX) entrapment efficiency (EE) of 97.79%, which is four times higher than that of pure mesoporous silica nanoparticles. The results of the research are very promising and silica and calcium phsophate combination can be further studied for drug delivery applications.

The use of calcium phosphate in drug delivery systems enables precise and localized delivery of therapeutic agents, minimizing systemic side effects and enhancing treatment efficacy. Calcium phosphate-based drug delivery systems have applications in various fields, including cancer therapy, bone regeneration, and targeted drug delivery to specific tissues or cells. Ongoing research continues to explore innovative strategies for utilizing calcium phosphate in drug delivery systems to advance personalized medicine and improve patient outcomes.

3.4 FUTURE PERSPECTIVE AND CONCLUSION

The book chapter provides a comprehensive overview of the types, structures, and applications of calcium phosphates in orthopedics. Through an exploration of their crystal structure and composition, the chapter elucidates the unique properties of these materials. The chapter concludes by highlighting the exciting potential for further exploration and development of calcium phosphates in orthopedics. Future research efforts should focus on advancing our understanding of the interactions between calcium phosphates and living tissues, as well as optimizing their properties for specific applications. This includes refining the design and fabrication of calcium phosphate-based scaffolds to enhance cell attachment, proliferation, and differentiation. Moreover, there is a need for continued investigation into the development of novel drug delivery strategies using calcium phosphates, aiming to improve targeted therapeutic delivery and efficacy. Overall, the versatility and promising clinical applications of calcium phosphates in orthopedics position them as an exciting and evolving field of research. Continued efforts in research and development hold the potential to revolutionize orthopedic treatments, leading to improved patient outcomes, enhanced tissue regeneration, and reduced complications associated with orthopedic interventions.

REFERENCES

1. V. Sokolova and M. Epple. Biological and medical applications of calcium phosphate nanoparticles. *Chemistry–A European Journal*, **27**(27):7471–7488, 2021.
2. Y. Hong, H. Fan, B. Li, B. Guo, M. Liu, and X. Zhang. Fabrication, biological effects, and medical applications of calcium phosphate nanoceramics. *Materials Science and Engineering: R: Reports*, **70**(3–6):225–242, 2010.
3. R. Sun, M. Åhlén, C.-W. Tai, É. G. Bajnóczi, F. de Kleijne, N. Ferraz, I. Persson, M. Strømme, and O. Cheung. Highly porous amorphous calcium phosphate for drug delivery and bio-medical applications. *Nanomaterials*, **10**(1):20, 2019.
4. S. Gautam, D. Bhatnagar, D. Bansal, H. Batra, and N. Goyal. Recent advancements in nanomaterials for biomedical implants. *Biomedical Engineering Advances*, **3**:100029, 2022.
5. M. Canillas, P. Pena, A. H. de Aza, and M. A. Rodríguez. Calcium phosphates for biomedical applications. *Bulletin of the Spanish Society of Ceramics and Glass*, **56**(3):91–112, 2017.
6. F. Ozdemir, I. Evans, and O. Bretcanu. Calcium phosphate cements for medical applications. In: Kaur, G. (eds) *Clinical Applications of Biomaterials*, pp. 91–121, 2017. Springer, Cham.
7. K. M. Zakir Hossain, U. Patel, A. R. Kennedy, L. Macri-Pellizzeri, V. Sottile, D. M. Grant, B. E. Scammell, and I. Ahmed. Porous calcium phosphate glass microspheres for orthobiologic applications. *Acta Biomaterialia*, **72**:396–406, 2018.
8. F. Carella, L. D. Esposti, A. Adamiano, and M. Iafisco. The use of calcium phosphates in cosmetics, state of the art and future perspectives. *Materials*, **14**(21):6398, 2021.
9. D. Bansal, D. Bhatnagar, D. Rana, and S. Gautam. Ferrite nanoparticles in food technology. In: J. P. Singh (Ed), K. H. Chae (Ed), R. C. Srivastava (Ed), O. F. Caltun (Ed), *Applications of Nanostructured Ferrites*, pp. 295–314. Elsevier, 2023.

10. S. Mofakhami and E. Salahinejad. Biphasic calcium phosphate microspheres in biomedical applications. *Journal of Controlled Release*, **338**:527–536, 2021.
11. A. Díaz-Cuenca, Diana Rabadjieva, Kostadinka Sezanova, Rumyana Gergulova, R. Ilieva, and S. Tepavitcharova. Biocompatible calcium phosphate-based ceramics and composites. *Materials Today: Proceedings*, **61**:1217–1225, 2022.
12. H. Zhou, L. Yang, U. Gbureck, S. B. Bhaduri, and P. Sikder. Monetite, an important calcium phosphate compound-its synthesis, properties and applications in orthopedics. *Acta Biomaterialia*, **127**:41–55, 2021.
13. O. Chan, M. J. Coathup, A. Nesbitt, C.-Y. Ho, K. A. Hing, T. Buckland, C. Campion, and G. W. Blunn. The effects of microporosity on osteoinduction of calcium phosphate bone graft substitute biomaterials. *Acta Biomaterialia*, **8**(7):2788–2794, 2012.
14. M. Bohner, L. Galea, and N. Doebelin. Calcium phosphate bone graft substitutes: Failures and hopes. *Journal of the European Ceramic Society*, **32**(11):2663–2671, 2012.
15. V. P. Galván-Chacón and P. Habibovic. Deconvoluting the bioactivity of calcium phosphate-based bone graft substitutes: Strategies to understand the role of individual material properties. *Advanced Healthcare Materials*, **6**(13):1601478, 2017.
16. C. W. Schlickewei, G. Laaff, A. Andresen, T. O. Klatte, J. M. Rueger, J. Ruesing, M. Epple, and W. Lehmann. Bone augmentation using a new injectable bone graft substitute by combining calcium phosphate and bisphosphonate as compositean animal model. *Journal of Orthopaedic Surgery and Research*, **10**:1–13, 2015.
17. J. Wu, B. Li, and X. Lin. Histological outcomes of sinus augmentation for dental implants with calcium phosphate or deproteinized bovine bone: A systematic review and meta-analysis. *International Journal of Oral and Maxillofacial Surgery*, **45**(11):1471–1477, 2016.
18. C. Pierre, G. Bertrand, C. Rey, O. Benhamou, and C. Combes. Calcium phosphate coatings elaborated by the soaking process on titanium dental implants: Surface preparation, processing and physical–chemical characterization. *Dental Materials*, **35**(2):e25–e35, 2019.
19. J.-M. Bouler, P. Pilet, O. Gauthier, and E. Verron. Biphasic calcium phosphate ceramics for bone reconstruction: A review of biological response. *Acta Biomaterialia*, **53**:1–12, 2017.
20. M. Parent, H. Baradari, E. Champion, C. Damia, and M. Viana-Trecant. Design of calcium phosphate ceramics for drug delivery applications in bone diseases: A review of the parameters affecting the loading and release of the therapeutic substance. *Journal of Controlled Release*, **252**:1–17, 2017.
21. S. Gautam, D. Bansal, D. Bhatnagar, C. Sharma, and N. Goyal. Synthesis of iron-based nanoparticles by chemical methods and their biomedical applications. In: P. Kumar, G. Kandasamy, J. P. Singh, P. K. Maurya. *Oxides for Medical Applications*, pp. 167–195. Elsevier, 2023.
22. C. Sharma, D. Bansal, D. Bhatnagar, S. Gautam, and N. Goyal. Advanced nanomaterials: From properties and perspective applications to their interlinked confronts. In: Kumar, R., Chaudhary, S. (eds) *Advanced Functional Nanoparticles "Boon or Bane" for Environment Remediation Applications: Combating Environmental Contamination Remediation and Management*, pp. 1–26. Springer, Cham, 2023.
23. Z. Tang, X. Li, Y. Tan, H. Fan, and X. Zhang. The material and biological characteristics of osteoinductive calcium phosphate ceramics. *Regenerative Biomaterials*, **5**(1):43–59, 2018.

24. J. Jeong, J. H. Kim, J. H. Shim, N. S. Hwang, and C. Y. Heo. Bioactive calcium phosphate materials and applications in bone regeneration. *Biomaterials Research*, **23**(1):1–11, 2019.
25. I. Denry and L. T. Kuhn. Design and characterization of calcium phosphate ceramic scaffolds for bone tissue engineering. *Dental Materials*, **32**(1):43–53, 2016.
26. S. Gomes, C. Vichery, S. Descamps, H. Martinez, A. Kaur, A. Jacobs, J.-M. Nedelec, and G. Renaudin. Cu-doping of calcium phosphate bioceramics: From mechanism to the control of cytotoxicity. *Acta Biomaterialia*, **65**:462–474, 2018.
27. J. Lu, H. Yu, and C. Chen. Biological properties of calcium phosphate biomaterials for bone repair: A review. *RSC Advances*, **8**(4):2015–2033, 2018.
28. A. Malhotra and P. Habibovic. Calcium phosphates and angiogenesis: Implications and advances for bone regeneration. *Trends in Biotechnology*, **34**(12):983–992, 2016.
29. M. Wang, Xi. Ge, Z. Cui, S. Wu, S. Zhu, Y. Liang, Z. Li, and W. W. Lu. Influences of strontium on the phase composition and lattice structure of biphasic calcium phosphate. *Ceramics International*, **47**(11):16248–16255, 2021.
30. L. He, G. Dong, and C. Deng. Effects of strontium substitution on the phase transformation and crystal structure of calcium phosphate derived by chemical precipitation. *Ceramics International*, **42**(10):11918–11923, 2016.
31. L.-H. Fu, Y.-R. Hu, C. Qi, T. He, S. Jiang, C. Jiang, J. He, J. Qu, J. Lin, and P. Huang. Biodegradable manganese-doped calcium phosphate nanotheranostics for traceable cascade reaction-enhanced anti-tumor therapy. *ACS Nano*, **13**(12):13985–13994, 2019.
32. P. S. P. Poh, D. W. Hutmacher, B. M. Holzapfel, A. K. Solanki, M. M. Stevens, and M. A. Woodruff. In vitro and in vivo bone formation potential of surface calcium phosphate-coated polycaprolactone and polycaprolactone/bioactive glass composite scaffolds. *Acta Biomaterialia*, **30**:319–333, 2016.
33. F. Kermani, S. Kargozar, S. V. Dorozhkin, and S. Mollazadeh. Calcium phosphate bioceramics for improved angiogenesis. In S. Kargozar (Ed), M. Mozafari (Ed). *Biomaterials for Vasculogenesis and Angiogenesis*, pp. 185–203. Elsevier, 2022.
34. M. Bohner, B. Le Gars Santoni, and N. Döbelin. β-tricalcium phosphate for bone substitution: Synthesis and properties. *Acta Biomaterialia*, **113**:23–41, 2020.
35. A. Lotsari, A. K. Rajasekharan, M. Halvarsson, and M. Andersson. Transformation of amorphous calcium phosphate to bone-like apatite. *Nature Communications*, **9**(1):4170, 2018.
36. J. Esguerra Arce, A. Esguerra Arce, Y. Aguilar, L. Yate, S. Moya, C. Rincón, and O. Gutiérrez. Calcium phosphate–calcium titanate composite coatings for orthopedic applications. *Ceramics International*, **42**(8):10322–10331, 2016.
37. S. Bose, D. Banerjee, A. Shivaram, S. Tarafder, and A. Bandyopadhyay. Calcium phosphate coated 3D printed porous titanium with nanoscale surface modification for orthopedic and dental applications. *Materials & Design*, **151**:102–112, 2018.
38. C. Combes and C. Rey. Amorphous calcium phosphates: Synthesis, properties and uses in biomaterials. *Acta Biomaterialia*, **6**(9):3362–3378, 2010.
39. H. Zhou and S. B. Bhaduri. The translatory aspects of calcium phosphates for orthopedic applications. In: L. Yang (Ed), S. B. Bhaduri (Ed), T. J. Webster (Ed). *Biomaterials in Translational Medicine*, pp. 37–55. Elsevier, 2019.
40. Y. Maazouz, I. Rentsch, B. Lu, B. Le Gars Santoni, N. Doebelin, and M. Bohner. In vitro measurement of the chemical changes occurring within β-tricalcium phosphate bone graft substitutes. *Acta Biomaterialia*, **102**:440–457, 2020.

41. G. Hettich, R. A. Schierjott, M. Epple, U. Gbureck, S. Heinemann, H. Mozaffari-Jovein, and T. M. Grupp. Calcium phosphate bone graft substitutes with high mechanical load capacity and high degree of interconnecting porosity. *Materials*, **12**(21):3471, 2019.
42. A. Kakar, B. H. Sripathi Rao, S. Hegde, N. Deshpande, A. Lindner, H. Nagursky, A. Patney, and H. Mahajan. Ridge preservation using an in situ hardening biphasic calcium phosphate (β-TCP/HA) bone graft substitute a clinical, radiological, and histological study. *International Journal of Implant Dentistry*, **3**:1–10, 2017.
43. W. R. Walsh, R. A. Oliver, C. Christou, V. Lovric, E. R. Walsh, G. R. Prado, and T. Haider. Critical size bone defect healing using collagen–calcium phosphate bone graft materials. *PloS One*, **12**(1):e0168883, 2017.
44. C. Kunert-Keil, F. Scholz, T. Gedrange, and T. Gredes. Comparative study of biphasic calcium phosphate with beta-tricalcium phosphate in rat cranial defects: A molecular-biological and histological study. *Annals of Anatomy-Anatomischer Anzeiger*, **199**:79–84, 2015.
45. C. Besleaga, B. Nan, A.-C. Popa, L. M. Balescu, L. Nedelcu, A. Sofia Neto, I. Pasuk, L. Leonat, G. Popescu-Pelin, J. M. F. Ferreira, et al. Sr and Mg doped bi-phasic calcium phosphate macroporous bone graft substitutes fabricated by robocasting: A structural and cytocompatibility assessment. *Journal of Functional Biomaterials*, **13**(3):123, 2022.
46. M. Touri, F. Moztarzadeh, N. A. Abu Osman, M. M. Dehghan, and M. Mozafari. 3D -printed biphasic calcium phosphate scaffolds coated with an oxygen generating system for enhancing engineered tissue survival. *Materials Science and Engineering: C*, **84**:236–242, 2018.
47. D. Bhatnagar, S. Gautam, H. Batra, and N. Goyal. Enhancement of fracture toughness in carbonate doped hydroxyapatite based nanocomposites: Rietveld analysis and mechanical behaviour. *Journal of the Mechanical Behavior of Biomedical Materials*, **142**:105814, 2023.
48. Y. Lin, S. Huang, R. Zou, X. Gao, J. Ruan, M. D. Weir, M. A. Reynolds, W. Qin, X. Chang, H. Fu, and H. H. K. Xu. Calcium phosphate cement scaffold with stem cell co-culture and prevascularization for dental and craniofacial bone tissue engineering. *Dental Materials*, **35**(7):1031–1041, 2019.
49. Y. Yang, Q. Yao, X. Pu, Z. Hou, and Q. Zhang. Biphasic calcium phosphate macroporous scaffolds derived from oyster shells for bone tissue engineering. *Chemical Engineering Journal*, **173**(3):837–845, 2011.
50. H.-X. Zhang, G.-Y. Xiao, X. Wang, Z.-G. Dong, Z.-Y. Ma, L. Li, Y.-H. Li, X. Pan, and L. Nie. Biocompatibility and osteogenesis of calcium phosphate composite scaffolds containing simvastatin-loaded PLGA microspheres for bone tissue engineering. *Journal of Biomedical Materials Research Part A*, **103**(10):3250–3258, 2015.
51. K. Thanigai Arul, E. Manikandan, and R. Ladchumananandasivam. Polymer-based calcium phosphate scaffolds for tissue engineering applications. In: A. M. Grumezescu (Ed). *Nanoarchitectonics in Biomedicine*, pp. 585–618. Elsevier, 2019.
52. S. de Lacerda Schickert, J. A. Jansen, E. M. Bronkhorst, J. J. J. P. van den Beucken, and S. C. G. Leeuwenburgh. Stabilizing dental implants with a fiber-reinforced calcium phosphate cement: An in vitro and in vivo study. *Acta Biomaterialia*, **110**:280–288, 2020.
53. C. Luo, S. Wu, J. Li, X. Li, P. Yang, and G. Li. Chitosan/calcium phosphate flower-like microparticles as carriers for drug delivery platform. *International Journal of Biological Macromolecules*, **155**:174–183, 2020.

54. B. A. J. A. van Oirschot, E. M. Bronkhorst, J. J. J. P. van den Beucken, G. J. Meijer, J. A. Jansen, and R. Junker. Long-term survival of calcium phosphate-coated dental implants: A meta-analytical approach to the clinical literature. *Clinical Oral Implants Research*, **24**(4):355–362, 2013.
55. C. Y. K. Lung, A. S. Khan, R. Zeeshan, S. Akhtar, A. A. Chaudhry, and J. P. Matinlinna. An antibacterial porous calcium phosphate bilayer functional coatings on titanium dental implants. *Ceramics International*, **49**(2):2401–2409, 2023.
56. H. S. Alghamdi, V. M. J. I. Cuijpers, J. G. C. Wolke, J. J. J. P. Van den Beucken, and J. A. Jansen. Calcium-phosphate-coated oral implants promote osseointegration in osteoporosis. *Journal of Dental Research*, **92**(11):982–988, 2013.
57. Q. Alkhasawnah, S. Elmas, K. Sohrabi, S. Attia, S. Heinemann, T. El Khassawna, and C. Heiss. Confirmation of calcium phosphate cement biodegradation after jawbone augmentation around dental implants using three-dimensional visualization and segmentation software. *Materials*, **14**(22):7084, 2021.
58. S. Anil, J. Venkatesan, M. S. Shim, E. P. Chalisserry, and S.-K. Kim. Bone response to calcium phosphate coatings for dental implants. In: A. Piattelli (Ed). *Bone Response to Dental Implant Materials*, pp. 65–88. Elsevier, 2017.
59. M. Prokopowicz, A. Szewczyk, A. Skwira, R. Skadej, and G. Walker. Biphasic composite of calcium phosphate-based mesoporous silica as a novel bone drug delivery system. *Drug Delivery and Translational Research*, **10**:455–470, 2020.
60. S. Gautam, J. Singhal, H. K. Lee, and K. H. Chae. Drug delivery of paracetamol by metal-organic frameworks (HKUST-1): Improvised synthesis and investigations. *Materials Today Chemistry*, **23**:100647, 2022.
61. R. F. Richter, T. Ahlfeld, M. Gelinsky, and A. Lode. Composites consisting of calcium phosphate cements and mesoporous bioactive glasses as a 3D plottable drug delivery system. *Acta Biomaterialia*, **156**:146–157, 2023.
62. J. Han, E.-K. Jang, M.-R. Ki, R. G. Son, S. Kim, Y. Choe, S. P. Pack, and S. Chung. ph-responsive phototherapeutic poly (acrylic acid)-calcium phosphate passivated TiO_2 nanoparticle-based drug delivery system for cancer treatment applications. *Journal of Industrial and Engineering Chemistry*, **112**:258–270, 2022.
63. A. Pylostomou, O. Demir-Oguz, and D. Loca. Calcium phosphate bone cements as local drug delivery systems for bone cancer treatment. *Biomaterials Advances*, **148**:213367, 2023.
64. A. Roy, S. Jhunjhunwala, E. Bayer, M. Fedorchak, S. R. Little, and P. N. Kumta. Porous calcium phosphate-poly (lactic-co-glycolic) acid composite bone cement: A viable tunable drug delivery system. *Materials Science and Engineering: C*, **59**:92–101, 2016.
65. Y. He, B. Zeng, S. Liang, M. Long, and H. Xu. Synthesis of ph-responsive biodegradable mesoporous silica–calcium phosphate hybrid nanoparticles as a high potential drug carrier. *ACS Applied Materials & Interfaces*, **9**(51):44402–44409, 2017.

4 The Essential Role of Calcium Phosphate in Bone Regeneration

Lidiya Sonowal and Sanjeev Gautam
Advanced Functional Materials Laboratory, Dr. S.S. Bhatnagar University Institute of Chemical Engineering and Technology, Panjab University, Chandigarh, India

4.1 INTRODUCTION

Humans and other vertebrates, including other animals, have skeletal systems made of bone, which is a hard, stiff connective tissue. It is an organic matrix, specialized cells, and inorganic mineral salts that make up a living tissue. In addition to providing structural support, bone also protects essential organs, promotes movement, stores minerals, and helps the body produce blood cells [1,2]. Cortical (compact) and trabecular (spongy or cancellous) bone are the two basic forms of bone. The outer, dense layer of bones, called cortical bone, offers strength and protection. Less dense but more metabolically active, trabecular bone develops a lattice-like structure inside of bones and is important in mineral exchange and blood cell synthesis [3].

Bone remodels itself continuously, with osteoclasts resorting to old bone and osteoblasts forming new bone to replace it. This remodeling procedure keeps bones strong, fixes micro-damage, and makes bones more resilient to shifting mechanical loads [4].

Bone regeneration is required to repair the structural integrity and functionality of a bone that has cracked because of trauma or damage or may be due to other defects. The gap between the shattered ends is filled in by the creation of new bone tissue, which enables appropriate healing and union. Techniques and methods for bone regeneration, including the use of bone transplants, scaffolds, growth factors, and stem cells, are intended to speed up the body's normal healing processes and promote the regeneration of healthy bone tissue. These methods are thus essential for improving the overall quality of life for those who have bone injuries or disorders, as well as for restoring bone form, strength, and functionality [5–7].

Calcium phosphate plays a vital role in bone regeneration. Materials made of calcium phosphate have osteoconductive qualities, which means they encourage

DOI: 10.1201/9781003360605-4

osteoblasts, the cells that make bones, to migrate, attach, and proliferate. Osteoblasts may easily form new bone tissue on calcium phosphate scaffolds, which encourages bone regeneration where a deficiency exists. Through a mechanism known as "bioactive bonding", calcium phosphate compounds have the capacity to establish a direct link with host bone tissue. The surface of calcium phosphate materials forms a layer of hydroxycarbonate apatite (HCA) when they come into contact with physiological fluids. This HCA layer creates a tight link and integration between the scaffold and the surrounding bone tissue by mimicking the structure and content of the mineral phase in bone [8–10].

Calcium phosphate materials, such as hydroxyapatite (HA) and tricalcium phosphate (TCP), have excellent biocompatibility, making them well-suited for bone regeneration applications. The mineral phase of calcium phosphate closely mirrors that of actual bone, creating an environment that is conducive to interaction with bone tissue. Due to their closeness, the scaffold and host bone can interact and integrate well, promoting bone regeneration [11, 12].

They are also bioactive, which means they can interact with the surrounding biological environment and cause cellular reactions. Such materials may develop a layer of hydroxycarbonate apatite (HCA) on their surface when they come into contact with body fluids. Additionally, materials made of calcium phosphate can be made to gradually deteriorate over time. The scaffold's regulated deterioration makes sure that it only offers temporary support until the freshly created bone tissue can take its place. The danger of long-term unfavourable effects is reduced by this controlled breakdown, which also encourages the rebuilding of healthy bone structure [13, 14].

4.2 BONE MINERALIZATION

The mineralization of bones depends heavily on calcium phosphate, especially hydroxyapatite. It gives bone tissue structural support, hardness, and mechanical stability. The body's mineral homeostasis is maintained by calcium phosphate, which also acts as a storage for vital ions [15]. Following section is an attempt to discuss the essential role of calcium phosphate in bone regeneration

4.2.1 HYDROXYAPATITE: THE PREDOMINANT CALCIUM PHOSPHATE IN BONE

Human bone and teeth are rich sources of hydroxyapatite (HA), a naturally occurring mineral form of calcium phosphate. With the chemical formula $Ca_{10}(PO_4)_6(OH)_2$, hydroxyapatite is a calcium phosphate compound. It has a crystalline structure with phosphate (PO_4^{3-}) and hydroxyl (OH^-) ions surrounding calcium ions (Ca^{2+}). These ions are arranged to provide hydroxyapatite its special characteristics, such as the capacity to adhere to bone tissue. Due to its biocompatibility, osteoconductivity, and resemblance to the mineral phase of natural bone, hydroxyapatite is frequently employed as a biomaterial in the context of bone regeneration and tissue engineering. To meet the needs of various applications, it can be synthesized in a variety of forms, including porous scaffolds, coatings, and nanoparticles [16–19].

In his study, Fang et al. attempted to create biologically-inspired hydroxyapatite micro-spheres from nanocrystalline hydroxyapatites in order to examine their curative capability and impacts on bone regeneration. The results suggested that the use of the hydroxyapatite micro-sphere can speed up the regrowth of alveolar bone. Additionally, other bone abnormalities may also benefit from this layout [20].

Bhatnagar et al. effectively infused carbonate into the HAp nanocrystalline in his work. The results demonstrated an increase in strength and toughness of the material thus indicating its further use as a biomaterial in the formation of implantable devices [21].

Frasnelli et al. synthesized strontium substituted hydroxyapatite nanopowders. The findings indicate that strontium substituted hydroxyapatite nanoparticles could be employed as an element of artificial bone alternatives to transport Sr to bone tissue and enhance its ability to regenerate [22].

4.2.2 MINERALIZATION PROCESS IN BONE

The deposition of inorganic mineral salts, predominantly hydroxyapatite (HA), onto the organic matrix of bone tissue is referred to as the mineralization process in bone [23]. It is a vital stage in the development of new bones and contributes significantly to the skeletal system's strength, hardness, and stiffness. The first stage of mineralization is nucleation during which amorphous calcium phosphate (ACP) is formed as a result of the combination of calcium and phosphate ions. For the following formation of HA crystals, these ACP clusters serve as the sites of nucleation. The creation of larger and more clearly defined HA crystals is caused by the addition of extra calcium and phosphate ions to the ACP clusters throughout the crystal growth process [24,25]. The collagen fibres become aligned with the HA crystals as they develop, creating a highly organized and mineralized bone matrix. This process takes place where active bone production takes occurred, in places known as mineralization fronts. The mineralization process is actively regulated by osteoblasts and osteocytes, guaranteeing optimum bone form and strength [26,27].

Thrivikraman et al. created a biomimetic method for the in vitro fabrication of a skeletal-like framework that mimics the nanoscale mineralization of 3D bone micro environments populated by osteoprogenitor, vascular, and neuronal cells **33**. The findings show that the suggested method permits extensive and virtually uniform mineralization of collagen hydrogels containing human mesenchymal stem cells (hMSCs) with ultrastructural organization and elemental composition similar to that of human bone [26].

Roschger et al. showed that the locations of bone remodeling and locations of de-novo bone creation at mineralizing sites of developing kids exhibit significantly diverse mineral characteristics and compositions. Contrary to popular belief, this suggests that the mechanism of bone mineralization may not be identical at different anatomical places. It was proposed that these variations result from different mineral precursor phase concentrations. This may be related to variations in the duration of the transit paths between the locations, which result in particular needs for long and short distance conveyance for mineral deposit [28].

Van et al. presents an effective approach for studying matrix-mineralization interplay in bone as a 3D cell-free in vitro system. It indicates that skeletal biomineralization is a physiochemical phenomenon that is matrix-driven and matrix-controlled and does not involve cellular activity [29].

4.2.3 ROLE OF CALCIUM PHOSPHATE IN BONE MINERALIZATION

In terms of minerals, calcium phosphate makes up the majority of bone. Crystals of the calcium phosphate compound hydroxyapatite (HA), which are formed during the mineralization process, grow and develop. The extracellular fluid of the bone matrix contains calcium and phosphate ions, which interact in a series of ways to cause the nucleation and development of HA crystals. The regulation of bone remodeling, a continual process of bone resorption and production, is influenced by calcium phosphate and the products of its dissolution. The calcium and phosphate ions that are produced by osteoclasts during bone resorption help to maintain mineral homeostasis. Calcium and phosphate ions are used to install new hydroxyapatite crystals during the ensuing bone production phase [30–33].

Zhi et al. created a calcium phosphate BCP biphasic bioceramic framework that exhibited favourable osteoconductive and osteoinductive characteristics by enhancing the component's chemical and physical attributes, and effectively mended significant segmental goat femur bone deformities. The results emphasized the role of the implantation mode and the importance of calcium phosphate bioceramic in bone regeneration [34] as depicted in Figure 4.1.

Duan et al. evaluated the ability of eight artificial CaP bone replacements to make bone, and discovered that different materials had different osteo-forming capacities. A certain pattern created by submicropores and micron-sized crystal grains was the essential catalyst for osteoinduction, and materials that released ions might increase inducing bone growth. It was concluded that instead of the existing notions that have been proposed such as protein adsorption, surface mineralization etc, the submicron-scale topography of the surface via specialized mechanotransduction may be the immediate trigger of osteoinduction in CaP bone analogues [35].

In an effort to provide the membrane the ability to stimulate osteogenesis and angiogenesis, Ye et al. created Sr-doped calcium phosphate/polycaprolactone/chitosan (Sr-CaP/PCL/CS) nanohybrid fibrous membrane through the inclusion of biologically active Sr-CaP nanoparticles into PCL/CS array. The results demonstrate that the Sr-CaP/PCL/CS nanohybrid electrically spun membrane has potential uses in guided bone regeneration (GBR) [36].

4.3 APPLICATIONS OF CALCIUM PHOSPHATE IN BONE REGENERATION

Numerous applications for calcium phosphate materials, particularly hydroxyapatite (HA) and tricalcium phosphate (TCP), exist in bone regeneration. Due to their outstanding biocompatibility, osteoconductivity, and similarity to the mineral

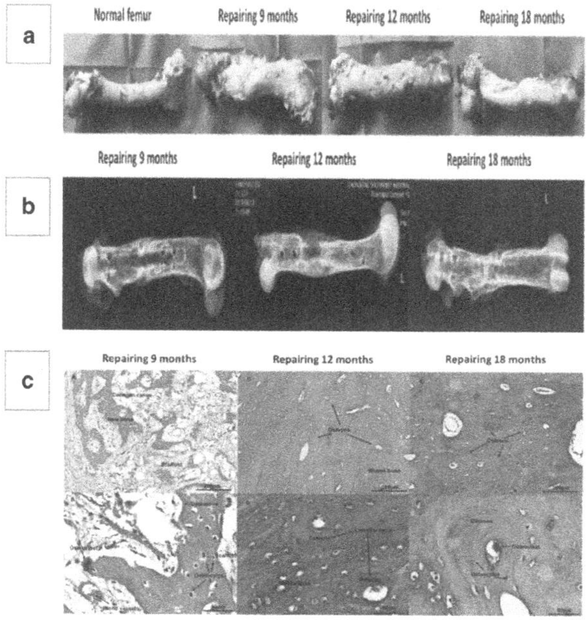

Figure 4.1 (a) Gross observation of goat femur in 9, 12, and 18 months of repairing. (b) The implant substance and recipient bone formed an intact bone link, as revealed by X-ray results. (c) The newly produced bone in the BCP scaffold from the mended femur by Zhi *et al.* [34].

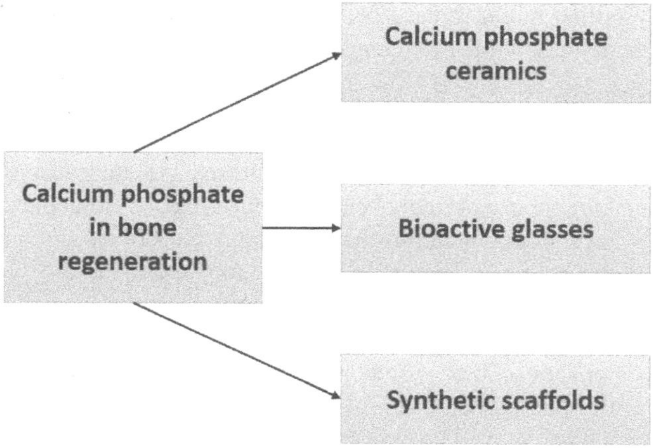

Figure 4.2 Illustration depicting applications of calcium phosphate in bone regeneration.

phase of natural bone, these materials are frequently employed in tissue engineering and regenerative medicine [37]. The following section is an attempt to discuss the major application of calcium phosphate in bone regeneration as represented in Figure 4.2.

4.3.1 CALCIUM PHOSPHATE CERAMICS

Ceramics are a family of inorganic materials that are noted for their extraordinary hardness, high melting temperatures, and chemical stability. They are made of metallic and non-metallic elements joined together through ionic or covalent connections. Ceramics that are predominantly made of calcium and phosphate components are known as calcium phosphate-based ceramics. These ceramics are ideally suited for a variety of biological applications, particularly in bone regeneration, because they closely mirror the mineral phase of normal bone [38–40].

Zhang et al. presented osteoinductive substances (Ca-P bioceramics) for osteo tissue frameworks with regulated deterioration rates, which is predicted to offer a regulated biodegradation pace to individuals requiring bone rejuvenation. The results demonstrated that an appealing option for customized skull bony tissue regeneration is 3D printable Ca-P bioceramics with a controlled decomposition rate [41].

Research led by Paulo et al. supported the theory that the dental material BCP, which is already utilized, has a protecting effect against zoledronate (ZOL) lethality. ZOL liberated from the bone may be captured if BCP is applied to the surgical site, reducing ZOL's bioavailability. This finding may indicate a possible Bisphosphonate Related Osteonecrosis of the Jaw (BRONJ) treatment option for patients receiving ZOL medication [42].

Investigations by Li et al. demonstrate that BCP ceramics with nano crystallinity can increase their biological activity, and a deeper comprehension of its effectiveness in directing bone formation will be crucial for uses of BCP nano ceramics in skeletal defect healing. The results further demonstrate that the porous BCP ceramic spheres with nanocrystalline might replace conventional osseous implants in purposes for repairing bone defects, while more long-term analyses are necessary [43].

4.3.2 BIOACTIVE GLASSES

A family of biomaterials known as "bioactive glasses" has the capacity to bind with live tissues, making them extremely beneficial in a range of biomedical applications. These glasses have special qualities that encourage bioactivity and interaction with the biological environment. They are made of inorganic materials, typically silica-based compounds [44, 45]. Calcium's incorporation in bioactive glasses has a number of benefits. First off, calcium plays a significant role in the production of natural bone, and its inclusion in bioactive glasses encourages the development of a positive contact with bone tissue. Calcium-based bioactive glasses begin the bioactive bonding process by creating a layer of hydroxycarbonate apatite (HCA) on their surface, which is analogous to the mineral phase of bone, when they come into contact with biological fluids. This HCA layer makes it easier for the glass to blend with the surrounding bone, aiding in bone healing and regeneration [46–48].

In his study, Capela et al. attempted to enhance bioactive glasses and glass-ceramics for clinical purposes and evaluated their bioactivity, biocompatibility, and antibacterial activities against *E. Coli* in vitro. The results concluded that raising

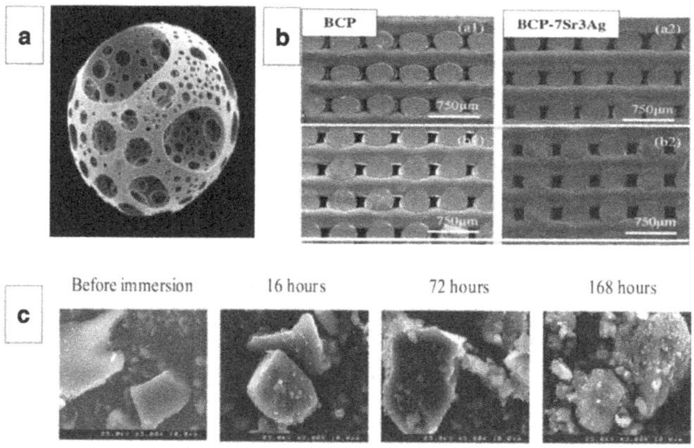

Figure 4.3 (a) Porous Glass microspore [51]. (Reprinted from Hossain *et al.* Copyrights Elsevier 2018.) (b) SEM images showing the interior microstructure of the BCP and BCP-7Sr3Ag scaffolds [59]. (Reprinted from Marques *et al.* Copyrights Elsevier 2017.) (c) Image of a glass sample taken before and after it was submerged in SBF [49]. (Reprinted from Capela *et al.* Copyrights Elsevier 2017.)

Ag_2O or reducing the dimension of particles tends to enhance the antibacterial effectiveness of the glasses toward *E. Coli* [49] as depicted in Figure 4.3.

An novel laser modification method was created by Menon et al. and the same was used on a copper doped bioresorbable calcium phosphate glass. This method made it possible to create precise micro-protrusion characteristics. It was demonstrated that the breadth and length of the generated extensions could be adjusted by adjusting laser settings and intricate exterior textures was obtained. The findings concluded that the metal-doped bio glasses can be surface texturized quickly, cheaply, and effectively, bringing up fresh possibilities for their use in the biomedical field [50].

In order to produce innovative permeable glass microspheres from calcium phosphate-based glasses and convey stem cells, Hossain et al. describes an affordable flame spheroidization procedure. The newly created unique microspheres have enormous promise for use in biological engineering and rejuvenation medicine [51] as presented in Figure 4.3.

In his investigation, Neto et al. derived Sr^-, Mg^-, and Zn-doped sol-gel bioactive glasses (BG) coated with biphasic calcium phosphates (BCP). The modified cuttlefish bone derived BCP scaffolds showed potential qualities, but additional evaluation of the *in-vitro* biological characteristics is required before considering applying them in bone tissue engineering applications [52].

4.3.3 SYNTHETIC CALCIUM PHOSPHATE SCAFFOLDS

By offering a temporary framework or structure to facilitate cell attachment, proliferation, and differentiation, scaffolds serve a crucial role in tissue engineering and regenerative medicine by directing the development of new tissue. They serve as models that replicate the extracellular matrix (ECM) and give cells a three-dimensional (3D) environment in which to develop and organdie [53, 54]. Scaffolds made of calcium phosphate have a number of benefits for bone tissue engineering. First, they have good biocompatibility, which means the body tolerates them well and they have no negative toxic or immunological reactions. This characteristic is essential for optimal healing and integration with the host tissue. Another advantage of calcium phosphate scaffolds is their ability to biodegrade over time. As new bone tissue forms, the scaffold gradually resorbs and is replaced by the natural bone, eliminating the need for surgical removal. The degradation products, primarily calcium and phosphate ions, contribute to the mineralization process and can further enhance bone regeneration [55–57].

In his investigation, Ramezani et al. intended to make connected porous biphasic calcium phosphate (BCP) scaffolds. The findings suggested that elevating the diopside concentration of the scaffolds enhanced their biological activity, biodegradability, and compressive toughness. In addition, compared to the BCP scaffold with zero weight percent diopside, the BCP with 15 weight percent diopside significantly boosted cell survivability and adhesiveness. The investigation indicates that skeletal tissue engineering applications may be possible for diopside/BCP scaffolds with enhanced biological and mechanical capabilities [58].

Three-dimensional porous calcium phosphate scaffolds were created by Marques et al. via robocasting biphasic powders that were both untreated and blended with Sr and Ag. The initial powders that were co-doped with Sr and Ag, increased the mechanical robustness of the scaffolds and gave them good antibacterial action. Additionally, human MG-63 cells were not adversely affected by the co-doping. Further, pre-osteoblastic multiplication was more successfully induced by the co-doped powder [59] as depicted in Figure 4.3

Xia et al. constructed a fresh Iron oxide based calcium phosphate scaffold (IONP-CPC scaffolds) using γ Fe_2O_3 and α Fe_2O_3 nanoparticles and seeded human dental pulp stem cells (hDPSCs) on it for skeletal tissue engineering. The findings reveal that the new CPC customized with IONPs has the potential to support skeletal restoration [60].

4.4 FUTURE PERSPECTIVE AND CONCLUSION

The field of bone regeneration has already been transformed by the use of calcium phosphate-based materials, which offer alternatives to conventional grafting techniques and enhance patient results. Researchers continue to explore and develop new techniques and materials to enhance bone healing and regeneration. Advanced biomaterials are being created by employing calcium phosphate-based substances to create materials that mirror the architecture and makeup of bone. Better mechanical strength, bioactivity, and a more effective bone regeneration process can all be provided by these biomaterials. Additionally, when calcium phosphate-based biomaterials are combined with 3D printing technology, it is feasible to produce patient-specific implants with exact structures and configurations. This individualized method can increase the efficiency of bone regeneration treatments and lower the possibility of implant rejection. Further, to speed up bone regeneration, researchers are looking into the use of calcium phosphate carriers for controlled medication administration. It is possible to offer localized and continuous release of growth variables, antibiotics, or other therapeutic agents into calcium phosphate-based materials, encouraging the best bone repair.

There is also a great promise of bone regeneration when stem cells and calcium phosphate-based biomaterials are combined. With these methods, significant bone abnormalities can be treated more thoroughly and successfully by generating functional bone tissue in a lab and transplanting it into the patient. Hence, Future research on calcium phosphate's use in bone regeneration is extremely promising.

In conclusion, multiple clinical scenarios have shown that calcium phosphate is effective and safe when used in bone repair. But for these materials and procedures to be even more optimized, continuous research and development is necessary. Developments in biomaterials, 3D printing, medication delivery methods, and tissue engineering could increase the effectiveness, dependability, and long-term success of bone regeneration operations, thereby enhancing patients' quality of life.

REFERENCES

1. G. Gautam, S. Kumar, and K. Kumar. Processing of biomaterials for bone tissue engineering: State of the art. *Materials Today: Proceedings*, **50**:2206–2217, 2022.
2. B. Q. Le, V. Nurcombe, S. M. Cool, C. A. V. Blitterswijk, J. D. Boer, and V. L. S. LaPointe. The components of bone and what they can teach us about regeneration. *Materials*, **11**(1):14, 2017.
3. A. N. Feldmann, P. Wili, G. B. Maquer, and P. Zysset. The thermal conductivity of cortical and cancellous bone. *European Cells & Materials eCM*, **35**:25–33, 2018.
4. D. B. Burr. Bone morphology and organization. In D. B. Burr (Ed), R. M. Allen (Ed), *Basic and Applied Bone Biology*, pp. 3–26. Elsevier, 2019.
5. L. Batoon, S. M. Millard, L. J. Raggatt, and A. R. Pettit. Osteomacs and bone regeneration. *Current Osteoporosis Reports*, **15**:385–395, 2017.
6. A. Ho-Shui-Ling, J. Bolander, L. E. Rustom, A. W. Johnson, F. P. Luyten, and C. Picart. Bone regeneration strategies: Engineered scaffolds, bioactive molecules and stem cells current stage and future perspectives. *Biomaterials*, **180**:143–162, 2018.
7. R. Dimitriou, E. Jones, D. McGonagle, and P. V. Giannoudis. Bone regeneration: Current concepts and future directions. *BMC Medicine*, **9**(1):1–10, 2011.
8. O. Suzuki, Y. Shiwaku, and R. Hamai. Octacalcium phosphate bone substitute materials: Comparison between properties of biomaterials and other calcium phosphate materials. *Dental Materials Journal*, **39**(2):187–199, 2020.
9. J.-M. Bouler, P. Pilet, O. Gauthier, and E. Verron. Biphasic calcium phosphate ceramics for bone reconstruction: A review of biological response. *Acta Biomaterialia*, **53**:1–12, 2017.
10. J. Jeong, J. Hun Kim, J. H. Shim, N. S. Hwang, and C. Y. Heo. Bioactive calcium phosphate materials and applications in bone regeneration. *Biomaterials Research*, **23**(1):1–11, 2019.

11. T. G. P. Galindo, Y. Chai, and M. Tagaya. Hydroxyapatite nanoparticle coating on polymer for constructing effective biointeractive interfaces. *Journal of Nanomaterials*, **2019**:6495239, 2019.
12. R. Taktak, A. Elghazel, J. Bouaziz, S. Charfi, and H. Keskes. Tricalcium phosphate-fluorapatite as bone tissue engineering: Evaluation of bioactivity and biocompatibility. *Materials Science and Engineering: C*, **86**:121–128, 2018.
13. I. Lodoso-Torrecilla, J. J. v. d. Beucken, and J. A. Jansen. Calcium phosphate cements: Optimization toward biodegradability. *Acta Biomaterialia*, **119**:1–12, 2021.
14. R. Khalifehzadeh and H. Arami. Biodegradable calcium phosphate nanoparticles for cancer therapy. *Advances in Colloid and Interface Science*, **279**:102157, 2020.
15. H. E. Karpen. Mineral homeostasis and effects on bone mineralization in the pretermneonate. *Clinics in Perinatology*, **45**(1):129–141, 2018.
16. A. Syauqina M. Zaffarin, S.-F. Ng, M. H. Ng, H. Hassan, and E. Alias. Nano-hydroxyapatite as a delivery system for promoting bone regeneration in vivo: A systematic review. *Nanomaterials*, **11**(10):2569, 2021.
17. N. Ramesh, S. C. Moratti, and G. J. Dias. Hydroxyapatite–polymer biocomposites for bone regeneration: A review of current trends. *Journal of Biomedical Materials Research Part B: Applied Biomaterials*, **106**(5):2046–2057, 2018.
18. A. Ressler, A. Žužić, I. Ivanišević, N. Kamboj, and H. Ivanković. Ionic substituted hydroxyapatite for bone regeneration applications: A review. *Open Ceramics*, **6**:100122, 2021.
19. S. Gautam, D. Bhatnagar, D. Bansal, H. Batra, and N. Goyal. Recent advancements in nanomaterials for biomedical implants. *Biomedical Engineering Advances*, **3**:100029, 2022.
20. C.-H. Fang, Y.-W. Lin, F.-H. Lin, J.-S. Sun, Y.-H. Chao, H.-Y. Lin, and Z.-C. Chang. Biomimetic synthesis of nanocrystalline hydroxyapatite composites: Therapeutic potential and effects on bone regeneration. *International Journal of Molecular Sciences*, **20**(23):6002, 2019.
21. D. Bhatnagar, S. Gautam, H. Batra, and N. Goyal. Enhancement of fracture toughness in carbonate doped hydroxyapatite based nanocomposites: Rietveld analysis and mechanical behaviour. *Journal of the Mechanical Behavior of Biomedical Materials*, **142**:105814, 2023.
22. M. Frasnelli, F. Cristofaro, V. M. Sglavo, S. Dirè, E. Callone, R. Ceccato, G. Bruni, A. I. Cornaglia, and L. Visai. Synthesis and characterization of strontium-substituted hydroxyapatite nanoparticles for bone regeneration. *Materials Science and Engineering: C*, **71**:653–662, 2017.
23. T. Hasegawa, H. Hongo, T. Yamamoto, M. Abe, H. Yoshino, M. Haraguchi-Kitakamae, H. Ishizu, T. Shimizu, N. Iwasaki, and N. Amizuka. Matrix vesicle-mediated mineralization and osteocytic regulation of bone mineralization. *International Journal of Molecular Sciences*, **23**(17):9941, 2022.
24. M. Edén. Structure and formation of amorphous calcium phosphate and its role as surface layer of nanocrystalline apatite: Implications for bone mineralization. *Materialia*, **17**:101107, 2021.
25. R. Gelli, F. Ridi, and P. Baglioni. The importance of being amorphous: Calcium and magnesium phosphates in the human body. *Advances in Colloid and Interface Science*, **269**:219–235, 2019.

26. G. Thrivikraman, A. Athirasala, R. Gordon, L. Zhang, R. Bergan, D. R. Keene, J. M. Jones, H. Xie, Z. Chen, J. Tao, and B. Wingender. Rapid fabrication of vascularized and innervated cell-laden bone models with biomimetic intrafibrillar collagen mineralization. *Nature Communications*, **10**(1):3520, 2019.
27. N. Dirckx, M. C. Moorer, T. L. Clemens, and R. C. Riddle. The role of osteoblasts in energy homeostasis. *Nature Reviews Endocrinology*, **15**(11):651–665, 2019.
28. A. Roschger, W. Wagermaier, S. Gamsjaeger, N. Hassler, I. Schmidt, S. Blouin, A. Berzlanovich, G. M. Gruber, R. Weinkamer, P. Roschger, E. P. Paschalis, K. Klaushofer, and P. Fratzl. Newly formed and remodeled human bone exhibits differences in the mineralization process. *Acta Biomaterialia*, **104**:221–230, 2020.
29. R. H. van der Meijden, D. Daviran, L. Rutten, X. F. Walboomers, E. Macías-Sánchez, N. Sommerdijk, and A. Akiva. A 3D cell-free bone model shows collagen mineralization is driven and controlled by the matrix. *Advanced Functional Materials*, 2212339, 2023.
30. L. Schröter, F. Kaiser, S. Stein, U. Gbureck, and A. Ignatius. Biological and mechanical performance and degradation characteristics of calcium phosphate cements in large animals and humans. *Acta Biomaterialia*, **117**:1–20, 2020.
31. C. Ma, T. Du, X. Niu, and Y. Fan. Biomechanics and mechanobiology of the bone matrix. *Bone Research*, **10**(1):59, 2022.
32. P Katsimbri. The biology of normal bone remodelling. *European Journal of Cancer Care*, **26**(6):e12740, 2017.
33. J. Kenkre and J. Bassett. The bone remodelling cycle. *Annals of Clinical Biochemistry*, **55**(3):308–327, 2018.
34. W. Zhi, X. Wang, D. Sun, T. Chen, B. Yuan, X. Li, X. Chen, J. Wang, Z. Xie, X. Zhu, K. Zhang, and X. Zhang. Optimal regenerative repair of large segmental bone defect in a goat model with osteoinductive calcium phosphate bioceramic implants. *Bioactive Materials*, **11**:240–253, 2022.
35. R. Duan, D. Barbieri, X. Luo, J. Weng, C. Bao, J. D. d. Bruijn, and H. Yuan. Variation of the bone forming ability with the physicochemical properties of calcium phosphate bone substitutes. *Biomaterials Science*, **6**(1):136–145, 2018.
36. H. Ye, J. Zhu, D. Deng, S. Jin, J. Li, and Y. Man. Enhanced osteogenesis and angiogenesis by pcl/chitosan/sr-doped calcium phosphate electrospun nanocomposite membrane for guided bone regeneration. *Journal of Biomaterials Science, Polymer Edition*, **30**(16):1505–1522, 2019.
37. R. G. Ribas, V. M. Schatkoski, T. L. do Amaral Montanheiro, B. R. C. de Menezes, C. Stegemann, D. M. G. Leite, and G. P. Thim. Current advances in bone tissue engineering concerning ceramic and bioglass scaffolds: A review. *Ceramics International*, **45**(17):21051–21061, 2019.
38. P. Dee, H. Y. You, S.-H. Teoh, and H. L. Ferrand. Bioinspired approaches to toughen calcium phosphate-based ceramics for bone repair. *Journal of the Mechanical Behavior of Biomedical Materials*, **112**:104078, 2020.
39. L. H. d. Silva, E. d. LIMA, R. B. d. P. Miranda, S. S. Favero, U. Lohbauer, and P. Francisco Cesar. Dental ceramics: A review of new materials and processing methods. *Brazilian Oral Research*, **28**:133–146, 2017.
40. Z. Chen, Z. Li, J. Li, C. Liu, C. Lao, Y. Fu, C. Liu, Y. Li, P. Wang, and Y. He. 3D printing of ceramics: A review. *Journal of the European Ceramic Society*, **39**(4):661–687, 2019.
41. B. Zhang, H. Sun, L. Wu, L. Ma, F. Xing, Q. Kong, Y. Fan, C. Zhou, and X. Zhang. 3D printing of calcium phosphate bioceramic with tailored biodegradation rate for skull bone tissue reconstruction. *Bio-Design and Manufacturing*, **2**:161–171, 2019.

42. S. Paulo, M. Laranjo, A. M. Abrantes, J. Casalta-Lopes, K. Santos, A. C. Gonçalves, A. B. Paula, C. M. Marto, A. B. Sarmento-Ribeiro, E. Carrilho, A. Serra, M. F. Botelho, and M. M. Ferreir. Synthetic calcium phosphate ceramics as a potential treatment for bisphosphonate-related osteonecrosis of the jaw. *Materials*, **12**(11):1840, 2019.
43. X. Li, T. Song, X. Chen, M. Wang, X. Yang, Y. Xiao, and X. Zhang. Osteoinductivity of porous biphasic calcium phosphate ceramic spheres with nanocrystalline and their efficacy in guiding bone regeneration. *ACS Applied Materials & Interfaces*, **11**(4):3722–3736, 2019.
44. F. Baino, S. Hamzehlou, and S. Kargozar. Bioactive glasses: Where are we and where are we going? *Journal of Functional Biomaterials*, **9**(1):25, 2018.
45. S. Kargozar, F. Baino, S. Hamzehlou, R. G. Hill, and M. Mozafari. Bioactive glasses entering the mainstream. *Drug Discovery Today*, **23**(10):1700–1704, 2018.
46. M. Tavoni, M. Dapporto, A. Tampieri, and S. Sprio. Bioactive calcium phosphate-based composites for bone regeneration. *Journal of Composites Science*, **5**(9):227, 2021.
47. F. Hajiali, S. Tajbakhsh, and A. Shojaei. Fabrication and properties of polycaprolactone composites containing calcium phosphate-based ceramics and bioactive glasses in bone tissue engineering: A review. *Polymer Reviews*, **58**(1):164–207, 2018.
48. M. Karadjian, C. Essers, S. Tsitlakidis, B. Reible, A. Moghaddam, A. R. Boccaccini, and F. Westhauser. Biological properties of calcium phosphate bioactive glass composite bone substitutes: Current experimental evidence. *International Journal of Molecular Sciences*, **20**(2):305, 2019.
49. M. Capela, D. Tobaldi, C. Oliveira, A. Pereira, A. Duarte, M. Seabra, and M. Fernandes. Bioactivity and antibacterial activity against E. Coli of calcium-phosphate-based glasses: Effect of silver content and crystallinity. *Ceramics International*, **43**(16):13800–13809, 2017.
50. D. Meena N. Menon, D. Pugliese, and D. Janner. Infrared nanosecond laser texturing of Cu-doped bioresorbable calcium phosphate glasses. *Applied Sciences*, **12**(7):3516, 2022.
51. K. M. Z. Hossain, U. Patel, A. R. Kennedy, L. Macri-Pellizzeri, V. Sottile, D. M. Grant, B. E. Scammell, and I. Ahmed. Porous calcium phosphate glass microspheres for orthobiologic applications. *Acta Biomaterialia*, **72**:396–406, 2018.
52. A. S. Neto, D. Brazete, and J. M. Ferreira. Cuttlefish bone-derived biphasic calcium phosphate scaffolds coated with sol-gel derived bioactive glass. *Materials*, **12**(17):2711, 2019.
53. M. Hippler, E. D. Lemma, S. Bertels, E. Blasco, C. Barner-Kowollik, M. Wegener, and M. Bastmeyer. 3D scaffolds to study basic cell biology. *Advanced Materials*, **31**(26):1808110, 2019.
54. M. P. Nikolova and M. S. Chavali. Recent advances in biomaterials for 3D scaffolds: A review. *Bioactive Materials*, **4**:271–292, 2019.
55. Q. Liu, W. F. Lu, and W. Zhai. Toward stronger robocast calcium phosphate scaffolds for bone tissue engineering: A mini-review and meta-analysis. *Biomaterials Advances*, **134**:112578, 2022.
56. F. Pupilli, A. Ruffini, M. Dapporto, M. Tavoni, A. Tampieri, and S. Sprio. Design strategies and biomimetic approaches for calcium phosphate scaffolds in bone tissue regeneration. *Biomimetics*, **7**(3):112, 2022.
57. T. Ghassemi, A. Shahroodi, M. H. Ebrahimzadeh, A. Mousavian, J. Movaffagh, and A. Moradi. Current concepts in scaffolding for bone tissue engineering. *Archives of Bone and Joint Surgery*, **6**(2):90, 2018.

58. S. Ramezani, R. Emadi, M. Kharaziha, and F. Tavangarian. Synthesis, characterization and in vitro behavior of nanostructured diopside/biphasic calcium phosphate scaffolds. *Materials Chemistry and Physics*, **186**:415–425, 2017.
59. C. F. Marques, F. H. Perera, A. Marote, S. Ferreira, S. I. Vieira, S. Olhero, P. Miranda, and J. M. Ferreira. Biphasic calcium phosphate scaffolds fabricated by direct write assembly: Mechanical, anti-microbial and osteoblastic properties. *Journal of the European Ceramic Society*, **37**(1):359–368, 2017.
60. Y. Xia, H. Chen, F. Zhang, L. Wang, B. Chen, M. A. Reynolds, J. Ma, A. Schneider, N. Gu, and H. H. Xu. Injectable calcium phosphate scaffold with iron oxide nanoparticles to enhance osteogenesis via dental pulp stem cells. Artificial Cells, *Nanomedicine, and Biotechnology*, **46**:423–433, 2018.

5 Self-Assembly and Nano-Layering of Apatite Calcium Phosphates in Biomaterials

Lidiya Sonowal and Sanjeev Gautam
Advanced Functional Materials Laboratory, Dr. S.S. Bhatnagar University Institute of Chemical Engineering and Technology, Panjab University, Chandigarh, India

5.1 INTRODUCTION

The intrinsic biocompatibility and osteoconductive qualities of apatite calcium phosphates have driven its use in bone tissue engineering, dental implants, and orthopaedic procedures [1]. Researchers have realized the significance of improving the structural traits and functionalities of these biomaterials in order to fully realize their promise [2]. Self-assembly and nano-layering have become effective methods for achieving this objective [3].

The spontaneous organization of apatite calcium phosphate nanocrystals into well defined structures without the need for outside assistance is one of the main benefits of self-assembly. Due to this process, hierarchical structures at the nanoscale are formed as a result of the material's inherent chemical and physical properties [4]. Due to their higher mechanical strength, biocompatibility, and bioactivity, self-assembled biomaterials are ideal for a variety of medical applications, including bone regeneration and dental implants [5]. Apatite calcium phosphates are nano-layered by carefully controlling the thickness and makeup of several layers of nanocrystals [6]. This method enables the nanoscale tailoring of the biomaterials' characteristics, which is essential for simulating the intricate structure of genuine tissues [7]. The layered technique influences the biomaterial's biodegradation rate, release of therapeutic compounds, and interaction with neighboring biological tissues in addition to improving the mechanical integrity of the biomaterial [8]. Furthermore, hybrid biomaterials with a synergistic combination of traits can be made by combining the self-assembly and nano-layering procedures. A localized and sustained release of therapeutic agents at the site of implantation, for example, can be made possible by

DOI: 10.1201/9781003360605-5

adding additional bioactive chemicals, such as growth factors or medicines, within the nano-layers [9].

In conclusion, the nano-layering and self-assembly of apatite calcium phosphates in biomaterials offer significant promise for the creation of cutting-edge and revolutionary medical devices and implants. Researchers now have the skills to create biomaterials with customized properties, improving tissue regeneration, lowering implant failure, and improving clinical outcomes across a range of biomedical applications. This is made possible by the capacity to fine-tune a material's structure at the nanoscale.

5.2 FABRICATION METHODS FOR APATITE CALCIUM PHOSPHATE BIOMATERIALS

Apatite calcium phosphate biomaterials can be developed via an array of techniques, each with its own benefits and uses. This sections attempts to discuss three most such common techniques and depict their advantages and disadvantages in Table 5.1.

Table 5.1
Various Advantages and Disadvantages of the Fabrication Methods for Biomaterials

Technique	Advantages	Disadvantages	References
Sol-gel synthesis	Versatility Homogeneity Control over composition	Slow process Potential impurities Limited mechanical strength	[10]
Biomimetic mineralization	Bioinspired properties Environmentally friendly Biocompatibility	Complexity Limited scalability Slow kinetics	[11]
Electrospinning	Nanofiber formation Mimicking tissue structures Drug delivery	Limited scalability Process complexity	[12]
Electrochemical deposition	Fast deposition Conformal coating Tunable properties	Energy consumption Substrate limitation Limited material options	[13]

5.2.1 SOL-GEL METHOD

A flexible and popular methodology for creating apatite calcium phosphate biomaterials, particularly hydroxyapatite (HAp) and tricalcium phosphate (TCP), is the sol-gel method. To produce the desired substance, the procedure entails multiple successive processes. A precursor solution is first created by dissolving calcium and phosphate sources, most frequently calcium nitrate or calcium acetate and ammonium dihydrogen phosphate or diammonium hydrogen phosphate, in a suitable solvent, like water or alcohol [14].

The calcium and phosphate precursors then interact with water molecules in the regulated hydrolysis reaction that follows in the precursor solution. After this hydrolysis, a network of amorphous gel containing calcium and phosphate species is created. The gel is then allowed to age for a predetermined amount of time, during which the gel network develops and stabilizes, resulting in the final apatite calcium phosphate material with the appropriate qualities [15].

Following ageing, the gel is dried to remove the solvent and water content, resulting in the production of a solid substance. Finally, the dried gel is calcined at high temperatures, typically between 600 and 1000 °C, to obtain the appropriate crystalline structure and improve the material's characteristics [16].

A polyacrylic acid sol-gel approach was reported by He et al. to create biocompatible RE-CaP luminous nanomaterials for cell bioimaging. This process was shown to be suitable for creating rare earth doped calcium phosphate nanocrystals (RE-CaP) as a cell bioimaging agent [17].

By using the sol-gel method, a unique three phased hydroxyapatite (HAp) and fluorapatite (Fap) glass ceramics was created by Jmal et al. and demonstrated the formation and development of hydroxyapatite nano-phase the results concluded that ceramics made of Fap-Hap glass exhibited mechanical qualities akin to those of enamel and dentin [18].

By using the alcoholic sol-gel method, a biphasic calcium phosphate (BCP) powder was efficiently created by Balbuena et al.. The sintering variables that were investigated in this work proved to be useful for encouraging effective granular consolidation and β-CPP phase removal [19].

5.2.2 BIOMIMETIC MINERALIZATION TECHNIQUES

A wonderful method for creating apatite calcium phosphate biomaterials that closely resembles the natural mineralization processes that take place in bones and teeth is to use biomimetic mineralization procedures. These techniques are based on biological systems, in which proteins direct the nucleation and development of apatite crystals by serving as templates [20].

One such method involves controlling the mineralization process using organic templates, such as proteins, peptides, or polysaccharides. These biomolecules have unique binding sites that draw calcium and phosphate ions, enabling the controlled and orderly production of apatite crystals. Researchers may alter the size, shape, and orientation of the apatite crystals, thereby affecting the properties of the biomaterial, by carefully choosing and manipulating these organic templates [21].

Enzyme-assisted mineralization is another biomimetic approach in which enzymes are used to manage the mineralization process. Enzymes have the ability to control pH, direct crystal formation, and regulate calcium and phosphate ion concentrations, resulting in biomaterials with increased bioactivity and biocompatibility [22].

Yet, another biomimetic technique is to incorporate bioactive ions, such as magnesium, strontium, or zinc, into the apatite structure during mineralization. By carefully incorporating these ions into the apatite lattice, which are known to promote bone formation and regeneration, biomaterials with improved osteogenic characteristics can be produced [23].

The conclusions of the investigation by Salama et al. demonstrated the effectiveness of CHI-g-P(SPMA) hydrogel as a framework to promote the development of sponge-like hydroxyapatite. The biomimetic mineralization study revealed that after 7 days of culture in SBF, rod-like hydroxyapatite with excellent homogeneity was produced [24].

In his study, Seredin et al. showed that a bioinspired nanocrystalline carbonate-substituted calcium hydroxyapatite (ncHAp), whose physical and chemical characteristics resemble to the natural apatite dental matrix, can form a biomimetic mineralizing layer on the exterior of dental enamel. This material is combined with an array of polyfunctional organic and polar amino acids [25].

To start biomimetic calcium phosphate mineralization through simulated bodily fluid, a green biomaterial made of cellulose grafted SPI was developed by Salama et al.. In order to build a long-lasting, biocompatible, and reasonably priced candidate scaffold for bone tissue creation, this work offers a green research approach [26].

5.2.3 ELECTROSPINNING AND ELECTROCHEMICAL DEPOSITION FOR NANO-LAYERED BIOMATERIALS

Two novel methods that show promise for the creation of nano-layered apatite calcium phosphate biomaterials are electrospinning and electrochemical deposition. These techniques provide fine-grained control over the nanoscale deposition of materials, enabling the development of biomaterials with improved characteristics and functions [27].

Through the process of electrospinning, nanofibers made of apatite calcium phosphate particles are created from a polymer solution or composite. A nanofibrous structure is created in this procedure by creating an electrically charged jet of the solution and collecting it on a grounded substrate. Researchers can create nanofibers with good bioactivity and mechanical strength by adding apatite calcium phosphate nanoparticles to the polymer solution. The extracellular matrix's structural similarity to the nanofibrous architecture encourages cell attachment, growth, and tissue regeneration [28].

On the other hand, apatite calcium phosphate layers can form in a regulated manner on conductive substrates thanks to electrochemical deposition. Apatite crystals are created when calcium and phosphate ions react on the surface of the substrate when an electric current is applied. The thickness and makeup of each layer can be precisely controlled using this approach to create tiny, nano-layered coatings. The resulting biomaterials have improved bioactivity and may be designed to release therapeutic ions or medications under precise control, which makes them perfect for implant coatings and drug delivery systems [29].

Liu et al. used layer-by-layer 3D printing and layer-by-layer electrospinning to create 3D-printed electrospun fibrous frameworks. These composites' 3D plastic structural space can easily and swiftly be changed in order to observe how the immune system is regulated. Here, 3D-M-EF scaffolds enhanced bone development in vivo by increasing the polarisation of M2 macrophages, which in turn encouraged osteogenic differentiation and angiogenesis [30].

By using biodegradable micro-nano electrospun fibres loaded with highly active conditioned medium of adipose-derived stem cells (ADSC-CM), Chen et al. proposed a novel regenerative therapy. By using emulsion electrospinning and protein freeze-drying technologies, ADSC-CM was successfully loaded into nanofibers with biological protection and adjustable sustained-release features.The loaded electrospun fiber's core-shell structure exhibits excellent pro-regenerative effects on skin and tunable sustained-release characteristics [31].

Electrochemical assisted deposition technology has been used by Cotrut et al. to effectively electrodeposit hydroxyapatite coatings on cp-Ti substrate. Denser coatings at a higher deposition temperature of 75 °C have a more compact layer consisting of smaller HAp crystals covering the entire surface. In light of this, it can be said that hydroxyapatite produced at a temperature of 75 °C represents a potentially promising material for coating metallic implants that will come into direct touch with human bones [32].

5.3 SELF-ASSEMBLY OF APATITE CALCIUM PHOSPHATES

As the definition goes, the self-assembly of apatite calcium phosphates refers to the spontaneous organization of nanocrystals into well-defined structures without the need for external intervention [33]. This section attempts to discuss the mechansims and applications of self assembly in biomaterials. The applications of self assembly has been depicted in Figure 5.1.

5.3.1 MECHANISMS AND FACTORS INFLUENCING SELF-ASSEMBLY IN BIOMATERIALS

Biomolecules, nanoparticles, or other components of the nanoscale interact with one another in fundamental physical and chemical ways to self-assemble in biomaterials. These interactions develop well defined structures and architectures on their own, without the need for outside assistance. The biomaterial's hydrophilic to hydrophobic area balance has an impact on how the material self-assembles.

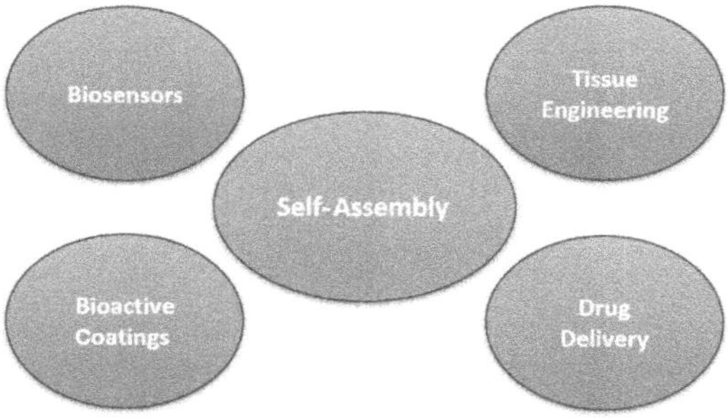

Figure 5.1 Illustrating the applications of self assembly in biomaterials.

Hydrophilic molecules like to interact with the watery environment, whereas hydrophobic molecules tend to agglomerate to reduce their contact with water. The organization of the biomaterial, which leads to the production of ordered structures, is driven by this delicate equilibrium [34].

Self-assembly is greatly aided by electrostatic interactions, which result from charged biomolecules or nanoparticles. The overall structure and stability of the biomaterial are further impacted by the attraction of components with opposing charges [35]. An other important variable that has an impact on self-assembly is the solvent selection. The organization and stability of the self-assembled structures may be affected by the composition and polarity of the solvent as well as its interactions with the biomaterial components [36]. Additionally, biomolecules or templates can serve as scaffolds by using template-directed assembly to direct the self-assembly of additional components all around them. Biomaterials with complicated and accurate structures are produced by this approach. In addition, the tendency of the system to decrease total energy and enhance disorder (entropy) can promote self-assembly. Components spontaneously arrange themselves into an advantageous configuration that uses the least amount of energy [37].

Mozhdehi et al. showed that the new creation of myristoylation substrates, which serve as peptide amphiphiles when recombinantly attached to an elastin-like polypeptide can control the hierarchical self-assembly of myristoylated peptide polymers [38].

Li et al. showed that encapsulated hMSCs' chondrogenesis is enhanced by self-assembled peptide hydrogels functionalized with N-cadherin mimetic peptide, and further explored the signalling processes and molecular mechanisms involved in this phenomenon. The outcomes serve as a guide for creating biomimetic biomaterials to support translational stem cell therapy. In the initial phase of chondrogenesis (day 3), chondrogenic gene expression is significantly greater in the N-cadherin mimicking peptide hydrogels (KLD-Cad) than in the KLD, KLD-Scr, and non-chondrogenic control groups. At late chondrogenesis (day 14), the type I collagen gene expression in the KLD-Cad group is much lower than in the KLD and KLD-Scr groups [39]. The chondrogenic expression has been depicted in Figure 5.2.

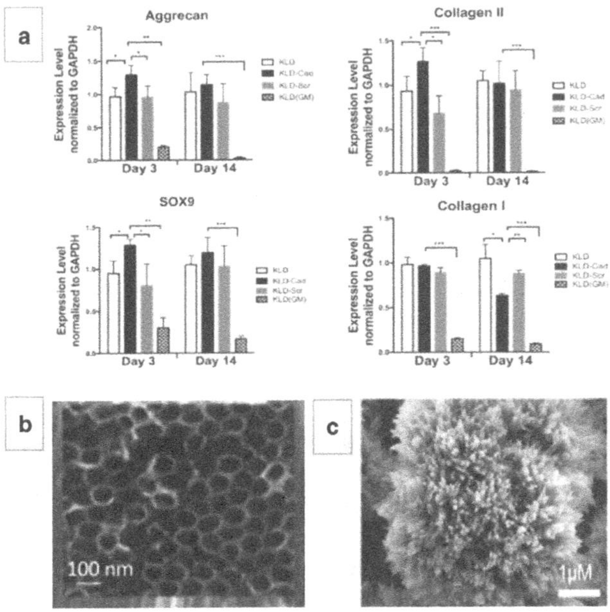

Figure 5.2 (a) Following 3 and 14 days of differentiation culture, the N-cadherin mimic peptide hydrogels showing chondrogenic gene expression [39]. (Reprinted from Li *et al.* Copyrights Elsevier 2017.) (b) Image of nanotubular titania at 100 nm. (c) HA deposition on nanotubular titania [46]. (Reprinted from Yazici *et al.* Copyrights Elsevier 2019.)

5.3.2 APPLICATIONS OF SELF ASSEMBLY IN BIOMATERIALS

Biomaterial self-assembly has a huge potential and is used extensively in a wide range of biomedical and materials science fields. Self-assembled biomaterials are used in tissue engineering, where they act as scaffolds for the regeneration of injured tissues and organs. These biomaterials encourage cell adhesion, proliferation, and tissue regeneration by acting as an artificial extracellular matrix. They are essential to the creation of artificial tissues, such as skin, cartilage, and bone substitutes [40].

Systems for delivering medications are a crucial application. Therapeutic substances, such as medicines or proteins, can be encapsulated within the core of self-assembled nanoparticles or micelles, offering an effective and controlled release platform [41]. Self-assembled biomaterials are used in the field of nanomedicine to transport imaging agents, enabling accurate and sensitive illness or biomarker detection [42]. Designing bioactive coatings for medical implants via self-assembly improves their ability to integrate with surrounding tissues. Additionally, self-assembled biomaterials are used in diagnostics as biosensors for identifying particular infections or proteins. The organized architecture can make it easier for target molecules to be recognized and bound, creating very sensitive and targeted diagnostic tools [43].

Studies by Mamuti et al. suggested that self-assembly assisted targeting helps make nanomedicine more location-selective at the target site. The molecular state difference causes faster clearance of other organs and deeper penetration at the diseased location. The emphasis was placed on molecular design, dynamic self-assembly, and the connection between structure and biological effects [44]. In his investigation, Liu et al. demonstrated that self-assembled DNA frameworks may accurately and adaptably encode the calcium phosphate (CaP) mineralization at the nanoscale [45].

In order to avoid bacterial infection at the implant material interface covered with a typical bioceramic, Yazici et al. designed a dual functional peptide that makes use of biomolecular self-assembly. This was accomplished by electrolytically depositing a calcium phosphate layer on nanotubular titanium. In a single step, the modified peptide self-assembled on the CaP coating. As a result, it was discovered that the implant surface considerably reduced bacterial adhesion when both gram-positive and gram-negative bacteria were present [46]. Images of nanotubular titanium and HA deposition on its surface has been depicted in Figure 5.2.

For the encouragement of dental pulp stem cells, Nguyen et al. suggested using a dentinogenic peptide that self-assembles into β -sheet based nanofibers that make up a biodegradable and injectable hydrogel [47]. Li et al. showed that elastin-like recombinamer (ELR) self-assembled fibrils can cause intrafibrillar mineralization. Amorphous calcium phosphates that had been stabilized by polyaspartate filtered into the self-assembled ELR fibrils selectively before crystallizing as hydroxyapatite nanocrystals with [001] axes parallel to the long axis of the fibril. As clearly established ELRs can be created and produced via recombinant technology, their molecular and structural characteristics can be adjusted. By analysing the ultrastructure of the self-assembled ELRs fibrils and their mineralization, we came to the conclusion that the most important element in causing intrafibrillar mineralization was not electrostatic interactions or bioactive sequences in the recombinamer composition, but rather the spatial confinement created by a continuum β-spiral structure in an unperturbed fibrillar structure [48].

5.4 NANO-LAYERING OF APATITE CALCIUM PHOSPHATES

Apatite calcium phosphates can be precisely controlled in their arrangement by the advanced production method known as nano-layering, which produces biomaterials with distinctive characteristics and functions. Herein, techniques for achieving nano material and their applications have been discussed.

5.4.1 TECHNIQUES FOR ACHIEVING NANO-LAYERING IN BIOMATERIALS

To produce nano-layering, several techniques are applied, each with its own special mechanics. An technique that is frequently used is electrochemical deposition, which involves submerging a substrate in a solution containing calcium and phosphate ions. Apatite nanocrystals form in layers as a result of the deposition of these ions onto the surface of the substrate under the influence of an electric current. Researchers can control the layer thickness and characteristics by adjusting process factors including applied voltage and current density [49]. Another method is called sol-gel deposition, in which a precursor solution containing calcium and phosphate sources is subjected to condensation and hydrolysis reactions, resulting in the formation of a gel network with calcium and phosphate species [50]. In template-assisted approaches, scaffolds or templates direct the layered growth of nanocrystals. On the surface of the template, biomaterial precursors are deposited or developed, where they align and organdie into several layers in accordance with the template's architecture. The intended nano-layered biomaterial is left behind once the template has been removed after the deposition is finished [51].

Investigations by Zhao et al. intended to determine the hydrolytic stability of 10-methacryloyloxydecyl dihydrogen phosphate calcium (MDP-Ca) salts in various pH settings with nanolayered and amorphous forms. Findings showed that while MDP-Ca salts in layered or amorphous structures are slowly hydrolyzed, nanolayers are eliminated by an acidic setting [52].

Manganese-calcium oxide nanolayers (NL-$MnCaO_2$) were created by Rashtbari et al. and characterized. It was investigated how synthetic particles behaved like enzymes and discovered a bifunctional nanozyme that serves as a peroxidase and catalase mimic. The outcomes showed that metformin inhibited the peroxidase-mimic activity of NL-$MnCaO_2$, and that this effect was amplified by increasing metformin concentration [53].

By examining the hydration, physicochemical characteristics, and biological performance of hydrated cements, Tu et al. aimed to determine the viability of using mineral trioxide aggregate (MTA) powder coated with polydopamine (PDA) in tooth and bone tissue regeneration. These findings show that dopamine works well as a covering material to support odontogenic differentiation and long-term human dental pulp cell culture on PDA-MTA substrates. Future research aimed at creating new biomaterials for dental uses will heavily consider this direction [54].

5.4.2 APPLICATIONS OF NANO-LAYERED STRUCTURES IN BIOMATERIALS

One of the main uses for nano-layered biomaterials is in drug delivery systems, where they allow for the regulated and precise release of medicinal chemicals. These biomaterials provide customized release kinetics by including several medications in distinct layers, improving therapy efficacy and lowering side effects [55]. Nano-layered biomaterials work well as scaffolds in tissue engineering to encourage cell adhesion, proliferation, and tissue regeneration [56]. They are also advantageous for dental implants because they enhance their integration with the surrounding bone tissue and have the potential to produce antibacterial compounds that fight infections. Medical devices with nano-layered coatings, such as implants and stents, increase biocompatibility and lessen negative reactions [57]. Nano-layered structures are also utilized in biosensors, providing a large surface area for biomolecule binding, leading to highly sensitive and specific detection of biomolecules or pathogens [58].

A layered nano-$SrFe_{12}O_{19}$-LDH/CS nanohybrid framework made of nano-Sr-LDH nanoplates arranged on a CS matrix and a CS matrix with a layered structure

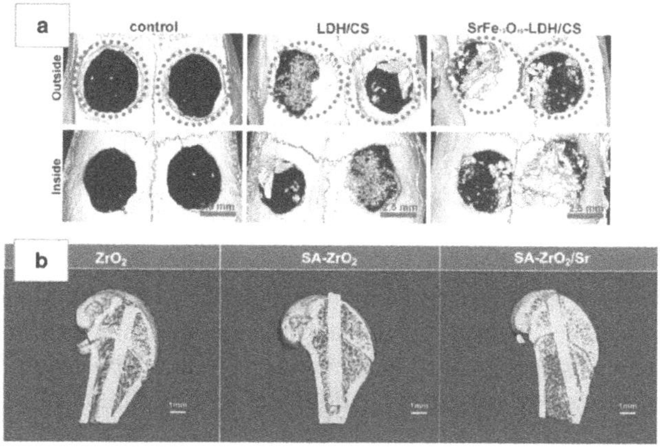

Figure 5.3 (a) A Micro-CT image showing new bone tissue forming in all three groups Ge *et al.* [59]. (Reprinted from Ge *et al.* Copyrights Elsevier 2022.) (b) Micro-CT scans of implanted 3D models of the surrounding bones [60]. (Reprinted from Li *et al.* Copyrights Elsevier 2021.)

was successfully by Ge et al.. The scaffold's stratified design encouraged the attachment and movement of bone marrow mesenchymal stem cells and macrophages, encouraged the development of the extracellular matrix (collagen fibres), and speed up the mineralization of freshly generated bone tissue [59]. The CT image of the new bone formed has been depicted in Figure 5.3.

By electrostatic engagement between the positive charges of the NPs and the negative charges of the graphene oxide (GO), the bone morphogenetic protein-2 (BMP-2)-encapsulated bovine serum albumin nanoparticles (NPs) were immobilized on the hydroxyapatite (HA) and tricalcium phosphate (TCP) by Xie et al.. TCP scaffolds were shielded against quick deterioration by GO nanolayers. Additionally, GO nanolayers enabled BMP-2 prolonged discharge and NP adsorption on these frameworks [61]. Li et al. used sandblasting, acid etching, and magnetron sputtering to successfully manufacture SA-ZrO2/Sr. The micro-surface structure, hydrophilicity, and surface roughness were all improved by the sandblasting and acid-etching processes [60]. The CT image of reconstructed model has been depicted in Figure 5.3.

Zhang et al. presented a straightforward, extensible, and repeatable method for fabricating 2D phosphate nanosheets by building a layered structure in situ using transition metal precursors and phytic acid (PTA). The interlayer carbon generated by the regulated burning of the organic groups in PTA serves to keep the layers apart while the phosphate is being formed, and when it is removed, ultrathin nanosheets with programmable layers are left behind [62].

5.5 FUTURE PERSPECTIVE AND CONCLUSION

Future developments in the field of biomedicine show enormous promise thanks to the self-assembly and nano-layering of apatite calcium phosphates in biomaterials.

These cutting-edge methods present a wide range of opportunities, and future research and technology developments are anticipated to broaden their scope and influence. The creation of more complex nano-layered scaffolds for tissue engineering has the potential to transform regenerative medicine. Researchers can create biomaterials that mirror the intricacy of original tissues by accurately manipulating the stacking of bioactive chemicals and growth factors, resulting in more successful tissue regeneration and organ transplantation.

It is anticipated that medication delivery systems would use nano-layered biomaterials' controlled release properties more widely. The capacity to customize medication release profiles to meet the demands of specific patients will become more and more valuable as personalized medicine gains traction, providing more effective therapies with fewer adverse effects. Additionally, the addition of nanoscale imaging agents to self-assembled apatite calcium phosphates will enable the creation of diagnostic tools that are extremely sensitive and focused. These biomaterial-based biosensors have the potential to revolutionize early illness monitoring and detection, resulting in better patient outcomes and more effective healthcare administration.

In conclusion, self-assembly and nano-layering of apatite calcium phosphates constitute a revolutionary direction in biomaterials research and development. In tissue engineering, medication delivery, diagnostics, and other fields, the capacity to precisely construct biomaterials with customized properties and functionalities has the potential to lead to substantial breakthroughs. As scientists continue to push these methods to their limits, we may anticipate amazing discoveries that will help millions of people around the world and influence the field of biomedicine. Adopting these cutting-edge methods would surely open up new avenues for personalized healthcare and regenerative medicine, ultimately enhancing the quality of life for countless people.

REFERENCES

1. F. Pupilli, A. Ruffini, M. Dapporto, M. Tavoni, A. Tampieri, and S. Sprio. Design strategies and biomimetic approaches for calcium phosphate scaffolds in bone tissue regeneration. *Biomimetics*, **7**(3):112, 2022.
2. D. Bhatnagar, S. Gautam, H. Batra, and N. Goyal. Enhancement of fracture toughness in carbonate doped hydroxyapatite based nanocomposites: Rietveld analysis and mechanical behaviour. *Journal of the Mechanical Behavior of Biomedical Materials*, **142**:105814, 2023.
3. A. Osaka. Self-assembly and nano-layering of apatitic calcium phosphates in biomaterials. In: Ben-Nissan, B. (eds). *Advances in Calcium Phosphate Biomaterials, Springer Series in Biomaterials Science and Engineering*, **2**:97–169, Springer, Berlin, Heidelberg, 2014.
4. S. Senapati, A. K. Mahanta, S. Kumar, and P. Maiti. Controlled drug delivery vehicles for cancer treatment and their performance. *Signal Transduction and Targeted Therapy*, **3**(1):7, 2018.
5. J. Chen and X. Zou. Self-assemble peptide biomaterials and their biomedical applications. *Bioactive Materials*, **4**:120–131, 2019.

6. N. Sezer, Z. Evis, S. M. Kayhan, A. Tahmasebifar, and M. Koc. Review of magnesium-based biomaterials and their applications. *Journal of Magnesium and Alloys*, **6**(1):23–43, 2018.
7. J. Cheng, H. Li, Z. Cao, D. Wu, C. Liu, and H. Pu. Nanolayer coextrusion: An efficient and environmentally friendly micro/nanofiber fabrication technique. *Materials Science and Engineering: C*, **95**:292–301, 2019.
8. K. Wijaya, E. Heraldy, L. Hakim, A. Suseno, P. L. Hariani, M. Utami, and W. D. Saputri. Synthesis and application of nanolayered and nanoporous materials. *ICS Physical Chemistry*, **1**(1):1–1, 2021.
9. Z. Xiao, Q. Zhao, Y. Niu, and D. Zhao. Adhesion advances: From nanomaterials to biomimetic adhesion and applications. *Soft Matter*, **18**(18):3447–3464, 2022.
10. S. G. Ullattil and P. Periyat. Sol-gel synthesis of titanium dioxide. In: Pillai, S., Hehir, S. (eds). Sol–Gel Materials for Energy, Environment and Electronic Applications, 271–283, Springer, Cham, 2017.
11. Y. Zhou, K. Liu, and H. Zhang. Biomimetic mineralization: From microscopic to macroscopic materials and their biomedical applications. *ACS Applied Bio Materials*, **6**:3516–3531, 2023.
12. Y. Li, J. Zhu, H. Cheng, G. Li, H. Cho, M. Jiang, Q. Gao, and X. Zhang. Developments of advanced electrospinning techniques: A critical review. *Advanced Materials Technologies*, **6**(11):2100410, 2021.
13. C. Li, M. Iqbal, J. Lin, X. Luo, B. Jiang, V. Malgras, K. C.-W. Wu, J. Kim, and Y. Yamauchi. Electrochemical deposition: An advanced approach for templated synthesis of nanoporous metal architectures. *Accounts of Chemical Research*, **51**(8):1764–1773, 2018.
14. K. Ishikawa and A. Kareiva. Sol–gel synthesis of calcium phosphate-based coatings–A review. *Chemija*, **31**(1):25–41, 2020
15. O. M. V. M. Bueno, C. Leonardo Herrera, C. A. Bertran, M. Angel San-Miguel, and J. H. Lopes. An experimental and theoretical approach on stability towards hydrolysis of triethyl phosphate and its effects on the microstructure of sol-gel-derived bioactive silicate glass. *Materials Science and Engineering: C*, **120**:111759, 2021.
16. D. Bokov, A. T. Jalil, S. Chupradit, W. Suksatan, M. J. Ansari, I. H. Shewael, G. H. Valiev, and E. Kianfar. Nanomaterial by sol-gel method: Synthesis and application. *Advances in Materials Science and Engineering*, **2021**:1–21, 2021.
17. W. He, Y. Xie, Q. Xing, P. Ni, Y. Han, and H. Dai. Sol-gel synthesis of biocompatible Eu^{3+}/Gd^{3+} Co-doped calcium phosphate nanocrystals for cell bioimaging. *Journal of Luminescence*, **192**:902–909, 2017.
18. N. Jmal and J. Bouaziz. Synthesis, characterization and bioactivity of a calcium phosphate glass-ceramics obtained by the sol-gel processing method. *Materials Science and Engineering: C*, **71**:279–288, 2017.
19. O. B. F. Balbuena, L. F. S. Paiva, A. A. Ribeiro, M. M. Monteiro, M. V. de Oliveira, and L. C. Pereira. Sintering parameters study of a biphasic calcium phosphate bioceramic synthesized by alcoholic sol-gel technique. *Ceramics International*, **47**(23):32979–32987, 2021
20. K. Shin, T. Acri, S. Geary, and A. K. Salem. Biomimetic mineralization of biomaterials using simulated body fluids for bone tissue engineering and regenerative medicine. *Tissue Engineering Part A*, **23**(19–20):1169–1180, 2017.
21. Q. Li, Y. Wang, G. Zhang, R. Su, and W. Qi. Biomimetic mineralization based on self-assembling peptides. *Chemical Society Reviews*, **5**:1549–1590, 2023.

22. R. Chen, X. Chen, Y. Wang, and B. Wang. Biomimetic metal–organic frameworks for biological applications. *Trends in Chemistry*, **5**(6):460–473, 2023.
23. S. Jiang, M. Wang, and J. He. A review of biomimetic scaffolds for bone regeneration: Toward a cell-free strategy. *Bioengineering & Translational Medicine*, **6**(2):e10206, 2021.
24. A. Salama. Chitosan based hydrogel assisted sponge like calcium phosphate mineralization for in-vitro BSA release. *International Journal of Biological Macromolecules*, **108**:471–476, 2018.
25. P. Seredin, D. Goloshchapov, V. Kashkarov, A. Emelyanova, N. Buylov, K. Barkov, Y. Ippolitov, T. Khmelevskaia, I. A. Mahdy, M. A. Mahdy, T. Prutskij. Biomimetic mineralization of tooth enamel using nanocrystalline hydroxyapatite under various dental surface pretreatment conditions. *Biomimetics*, **7**(3):111, 2022.
26. A. Salama, N. Shukry, A. El-Gendy, and M. El-Sakhawy. Bioactive cellulose grafted soy protein isolate towards biomimetic calcium phosphate mineralization. *Industrial Crops and Products*, **95**:170–174, 2017.
27. L. E. Beckett, J. T. Lewis, T. K. Tonge, and L. T. J. Korley. Enhancement of the mechanical properties of hydrogels with continuous fibrous reinforcement. *ACS Biomaterials Science & Engineering*, **6**(10):5453–5473, 2020.
28. P. J. Rivero, D. M. Redin, and R. J. Rodríguez. Electrospinning: A powerful tool to improve the corrosion resistance of metallic surfaces using nanofibrous coatings. *Metals*, **10**(3):350, 2020.
29. M. B. Kannan. Electrochemical deposition of calcium phosphates on magnesium and its alloys for improved biodegradation performance: A review. *Surface and Coatings Technology*, **301**:36–41, 2016.
30. X. Liu, M. Chen, J. Luo, H. Zhao, X. Zhou, Q. Gu, H. Yang, X. Zhu, W. Cui, and Q. Shi. Immunopolarization-regulated 3D printed-electrospun fibrous scaffolds for bone regeneration. *Biomaterials*, **276**:121037, 2021.
31. L. Chen, L. Cheng, Z. Wang, J. Zhang, X. Mao, Z. Liu, Y. Zhang, W. Cui, and X. Sun. Conditioned medium-electrospun fiber biomaterials for skin regeneration. *Bioactive Materials*, **6**(2):361–374, 2021.
32. C. M. Cotrut, A. Vladescu, M. Dinu, and D. M. Vranceanu. Influence of deposition temperature on the properties of hydroxyapatite obtained by electrochemical assisted deposition. *Ceramics International*, **44**(1):669–677, 2018.
33. A. Levin, T. A. Hakala, L. Schnaider, G. J. L. Bernardes, E. Gazit, and T. P. J. Knowles. Biomimetic peptide self-assembly for functional materials. *Nature Reviews Chemistry*, **4**(11):615–634, 2020.
34. R. J. Betush, J. M. Urban, and B. L. Nilsson. Balancing hydrophobicity and sequence pattern to influence self-assembly of amphipathic peptides. *Peptide Science*, **110**(1):e23099, 2018.
35. J. Heo, M. Choi, and J. Hong. Facile surface modification of polyethylene film via spray-assisted layer-by-layer self-assembly of graphene oxide for oxygen barrier properties. *Scientific Reports*, **9**(1):2754, 2019.
36. L. I. Atanase and G. Riess. Self-assembly of block and graft copolymers in organic solvents: An overview of recent advances. *Polymers*, **10**(1):62, 2018.
37. J. Zhou, X. Wu, Y. Chen, C. Yang, R. Yang, J. Tan, Y. Liu, L. Qiu, and H. Cheng. 3D printed template-directed assembly of multiscale graphene structures. *Advanced Functional Materials*, **32**(18):2105879, 2022.

38. D. Mozhdehi, K. M. Luginbuhl, J. R. Simon, M. Dzuricky, R. Berger, H. S. Varol, F. Huang, K. L. Buehne, N. R. Mayne, I. Weitzhandler, M. Bonn. Genetically encoded lipid–polypeptide hybrid biomaterials that exhibit temperature triggered hierarchical self-assembly. *Nature Chemistry*, **10**(5):496–505, 2018.
39. R. Li, J. Xu, D. Siu Hong Wong, J. Li, P. Zhao, and L. Bian. Self-assembled n-cadherin mimetic peptide hydrogels promote the chondrogenesis of mesenchymal stem cells through inhibition of canonical wnt/β-catenin signaling. *Biomaterials*, **145**:33–43, 2017.
40. P. Yu, R. Bao, X. Shi, W. Yang, and M. Yang. Self-assembled high-strength hydroxyapatite/graphene oxide/chitosan composite hydrogel for bone tissue engineering. *Carbohydrate Polymers*, **155**:507–515, 2017.
41. J. K. Sahoo, M. A. VandenBerg, and M. J. Webber. Injectable network biomaterials via molecular or colloidal self-assembly. *Advanced Drug Delivery Reviews*, **127**:185–207, 2018.
42. P. Zou, W. Chen, T. Sun, Y. Gao, L. Li, and H. Wang. Recent advances: Peptides and self-assembled peptide-nanosystems for antimicrobial therapy and diagnosis. *Biomaterials Science*, **8**(18):4975–4996, 2020.
43. C. M. A. Brett. Perspectives and challenges for self-assembled layer-by-layer biosensor and biomaterial architectures. *Current Opinion in Electrochemistry*, **12**:21–26, 2018.
44. M. Mamuti, R. Zheng, H. An, and H. Wang. In vivo self-assembled nanomedicine. *Nano Today*, **36**:101036, 2021.
45. X. Liu, X. Jing, P. Liu, M. Pan, Z. Liu, X. Dai, J. Lin, Q. Li, F. Wang, S. Yang, L. Wang. DNA framework-encoded mineralization of calcium phosphate. *Chem*, **6**(2):472–485, 2020.
46. H. Yazici, G. Habib, K. Boone, M. Urgen, F. S. Utku, and C. Tamerler. Self-assembling antimicrobial peptides on nanotubular titanium surfaces coated with calcium phosphate for local therapy. *Materials Science and Engineering: C*, **94**:333–343, 2019.
47. P. K. Nguyen, W. Gao, S. D. Patel, Z. Siddiqui, S. Weiner, E. Shimizu, B. Sarkar, and V. A. Kumar. Self-assembly of a dentinogenic peptide hydrogel. *ACS Omega*, **3**(6):5980–5987, 2018.
48. Y. Li, J. C. Rodriguez-Cabello, and C. Aparicio. Intrafibrillar mineralization of self-assembled elastin-like recombinamer fibrils. *ACS Applied Materials & Interfaces*, **9**(7):5838–5846, 2017.
49. D. Tonelli, E. Scavetta, and I. Gualandi. Electrochemical deposition of nanomaterials for electrochemical sensing. *Sensors*, **19**(5):1186, 2019.
50. S. Grigoriev, C. Sotova, A. Vereschaka, V. Uglov, and N. Cherenda. Modifying coatings for medical implants made of titanium alloys. *Metals*, **13**(4):718, 2023.
51. M. Sahebalzamani, M. Ziminska, H. O. McCarthy, T. J. Levingstone, N. J. Dunne, and A. R. Hamilton. Advancing bone tissue engineering one layer at a time: A layer-by-layer assembly approach to 3D bone scaffold materials. *Biomaterials Science*, **10**(11):2734–2758, 2022.
52. Q. Zhao, Y. Gao, X. Jin, F. Han, K. Chen, and C. Chen. Influence of acidic environment on hydrolytic stability of MDP-Ca salts with nanolayered and amorphous structures. *International Journal of Nanomedicine*, **17**:1695–1709, 2022.
53. S. Rashtbari, G. Dehghan, S. Khataee, M. Amini, and A. Khataee. Dual enzymes-mimic activity of nanolayered manganese-calcium oxide for fluorometric determination of metformin. *Chemosphere*, **291**:133063, 2022.

54. M.-G. Tu, C.-C. Ho, T.-T. Hsu, T.-H. Huang, M.-J. Lin, and M.-Y. Shie. Mineral trioxide aggregate with mussel-inspired surface nanolayers for stimulating odontogenic differentiation of dental pulp cells. *Journal of Endodontics*, 44(6):963–970, 2018.
55. A. Sarode, A. Annapragada, J. Guo, and S. Mitragotri. Layered self-assemblies for controlled drug delivery: A translational overview. *Biomaterials*, **242**:119929, 2020.
56. P. Kumar, Y. E. Choonara, R. A. Khan, and V. Pillay. The chemo-biological outreach of nano-biomaterials: Implications for tissue engineering and regenerative medicine. *Current Pharmaceutical Design*, **23**(24):3538–3549, 2017.
57. A. Han, J. K. H. Tsoi, C. Y. K. Lung, and J. P. Matinlinna. An introduction of biological performance of zirconia with different surface characteristics: A review. *Dental Materials Journal*, **39**(4):523–530, 2020.
58. X. Ma, W. Ding, C. Wang, H. Wu, X. Tian, M. Lyu, and S. Wang. Dnazyme biosensors for the detection of pathogenic bacteria. *Sensors and Actuators B: Chemical*, **331**:129422, 2021.
59. Y.-W. Ge, Z.-H. Fan, Q.-F. Ke, Y.-P. Guo, C.-Q. Zhang, and W.-T. Jia. $SrFe_{12}O_{19}$-doped nano-layered double hydroxide/chitosan layered scaffolds with a nacremimetic architecture guide in situ bone ingrowth and regulate bone homeostasis. *Materials Today Bio*, **16**:100362, 2022.
60. L. Li, L. Yao, H. Wang, X. Shen, W. Lou, C. Huang, and G. Wu. Magnetron sputtering of strontium nanolayer on zirconia implant to enhance osteogenesis. *Materials Science and Engineering: C*, **127**:112191, 2021.
61. C. Xie, H. Sun, K. Wang, W. Zheng, X. Lu, and F. Ren. Graphene oxide nanolayers as nanoparticle anchors on biomaterial surfaces with nanostructures and charge balance for bone regeneration. *Journal of Biomedical Materials Research Part A*, **105**(5):1311–1323, 2017.
62. W. Zhang, P. Oulego, S. K. Sharma, X.-L. Yang, L.-J. Li, G. Rothenberg, and N. R. Shiju. Self-exfoliated synthesis of transition metal phosphate nanolayers for selective aerobic oxidation of ethyl lactate to ethyl pyruvate. *ACS Catalysis*, **10**(7):3958–3967, 2020.

6 Characterization of Calcium Phosphate Using Vibrational Spectroscopies

Priyal Singhal, Sanjeev Gautam and G.S.S. Saini
Advanced Functional Materials Laboratory, Dr. S.S. Bhatnagar University Institute of Chemical Engineering and Technology, Panjab University, Chandigarh, India

6.1 INTRODUCTION

Calcium phosphate materials hold significant importance in various scientific and biomedical fields due to their wide range of applications, including bone tissue engineering, drug delivery systems, and dental implants. Understanding the composition and properties of these materials is crucial for their successful utilization. Vibrational spectroscopies, such as Raman spectroscopy, and Fourier Transform Infrared (FTIR) spectroscopy, have emerged as powerful techniques for the characterization of calcium phosphate compounds. This chapter provides an in-depth analysis of the characterization of calcium phosphate using vibrational spectroscopies.

One of the most extensively studied and widely used forms of calcium phosphate available in the market include hydroxyapatite, tri-calcium, tetra-calcium, and biphasic calcium phosphate. These CaP ceramics have garnered significant attention in various scientific and clinical settings due to its compatibility and minimal toxicity with living tissues. CaP materials are considered highly bioactive due to their chemical similarity to the mineral component of natural bone. When CaP ceramics come into contact with bone cells, they undergo a process known as surface dissolution or ion exchange. This process leads to the release of calcium (Ca^{2+}) and phosphate (PO_4^{3-}) ions, which mimic the natural mineral components found in bone. The released ions form a strong chemical bond with surrounding tissues, promoting osseointegration and facilitating the regeneration of damaged bone.

FTIR spectroscopy is used to identify various spectral characteristics of the sample. The obtained spectrogram, also known as a spectrum, displays the intensity of the infrared (IR) radiation absorbed by the sample at different wavelengths or wave numbers. The spectrum is typically represented as a plot with the intensity of absorption on the y-axis and the wave number (which is the reciprocal of wavelength)

DOI: 10.1201/9781003360605-6

on the x-axis. By analyzing the spectrum, we can extract significant information about the sample. The spectrum reveals the location of peaks, which are specific absorption bands corresponding to molecular vibrations within the sample. Each peak represents a particular chemical group or functional unit in the sample. By identifying the location of these peaks, we can gain insights into the presence of specific chemical bonds or molecular structures within the CaP material. Additionally, the intensity of the peaks in the spectrum provides information about the abundance or concentration of the corresponding chemical groups. Higher intensities indicate a higher concentration of the associated functional groups or molecular vibrations. This allows us to assess the relative proportions or composition of different components within the CaP sample. Broader peaks suggest greater molecular disorder or structural variations within the sample. By analyzing the spectral peaks, it is possible to gain insights into the chemical composition, functional groups, and molecular structure of the CaP material under investigation [1].

Different phases, such as HAp and TCP, exhibit distinct infrared absorption patterns, allowing for their identification and quantification within a sample. Furthermore, FTIR spectroscopy offers practical advantages as an everyday approach for CaP analysis. Compared to other techniques, it is relatively quick and easy to perform, making it a convenient tool for routine characterization.

Tetracalcium phosphate (TTCP), represented by the chemical formula $Ca_4(PO_4)_2O$, is a calcium phosphate compound that stands out among other calcium phosphates due to its highest calcium-to-phosphorus (Ca/P) ratio of 2. The Ca/P ratio is a critical parameter that influences the properties and behavior of calcium phosphate compounds. In the case of TTCP, its elevated Ca/P ratio results in a higher basicity, meaning it has a greater alkaline nature compared to other calcium phosphates. TTCP has the ability to interact favorably with biological systems without causing harmful effects or adverse reactions.

The high biocompatibility of TTCP is of great interest in the field of biomaterials and tissue engineering. It suggests that TTCP has the potential to be utilized in various biomedical applications, such as the development of bone grafts, dental materials, and orthopedic implants.

When basic TTCP and acidic DCPA are combined with water, pure hydroxyapatite ($Ca_5(PO_4)_3OH$) is formed [2].

$$Ca_4(PO_4)_2O + CaHPO_4.H_2O \rightarrow Ca_5(PO_4)_3OH \tag{6.1}$$

In this reaction, TTCP acts as the basic component, while DCPA serves as the acidic component. When these two components are mixed with water, a chemical transformation occurs, resulting in the formation of pure hydroxyapatite. This reaction sparked the creation of a promising material for dental and orthopedic applications—the calcium phosphate cement (CPC). The self-setting property of calcium phosphate cement is highly desirable in various biomedical applications, particularly in dentistry and orthopedics. Unlike traditional cements that require external setting agents, such as heat or additional chemicals, self-setting cements solidify independently when exposed to physiological conditions or moisture. The solidified cement provides structural support and acts as a scaffold for new bone formation.

Table 6.1
Different Forms of Calcium Phosphate [3,4]

Name	Abbreviation	Ca/P
Amorphous calcium phosphate	ACP	1.2–2.2
Octacalcium phosphate	OCP	1.33
β-tricalcium phosphate	β-TCP	1.50
α-tricalcium phosphate	α-TCP	1.50
Hydroxyapatite	HAp	1.67
Tetracalcium phosphate	TTCP	2

Moreover, the absence of any by-products in the reaction ensures that the resulting cement is pure and free from potentially harmful substances.

Both Raman and FTIR spectroscopy can be employed to characterize calcium phosphate. Raman spectroscopy measures the inelastic scattering of light, providing information about the vibrational modes and crystal structure of materials. FTIR spectroscopy, on the other hand, analyzes the absorption of infrared radiation, revealing the presence of specific chemical bonds and functional groups. Commonly used forms of calcium phosphate are represented in Table 6.1.

6.2 SYNTHESIS AND PREPARATION METHODS

The synthesis and preparation of calcium phosphate (CaP) materials are crucial steps in their characterization and subsequent analysis using vibrational spectroscopies. Various methods have been developed to synthesize CaP compounds with controlled compositions, crystallinity, and morphologies.

6.2.1 WET CHEMICAL PRECIPITATION METHOD

In this method, a calcium source (e.g., calcium nitrate, calcium chloride,calcium hydroxide) and a phosphate source (e.g., ammonium phosphate, sodium phosphate, orthophosphoric acid) are mixed under controlled conditions, such as pH and temperature. The reaction between the calcium and phosphate ions leads to the formation of CaP precipitates. The obtained precipitates can be further processed to obtain desired CaP products.

The wet chemical precipitation method offers several advantages for synthesizing calcium phosphates. First, the synthesis process is relatively simple and quick. The precipitation reaction progresses efficiently, allowing for the formation of calcium phosphates in a relatively short period. This is beneficial in laboratory settings where timely synthesis is desired for further characterization and analysis. The precursors used for the synthesis of calcium phosphate are usually accessible and cost-effective [5]. Additionally, the wet chemical precipitation method has the benefit of yielding water as the only by-product. This is advantageous from an environmental perspective, as the synthesis process does not generate any harmful or undesirable by-products.

6.2.2 SOL-GEL METHOD

In this method, a precursor solution containing a calcium source and a phosphate source is prepared. Calcium precursors can include calcium nitrate, calcium chloride, or calcium alkoxides, while phosphate sources may include ammonium phosphate or sodium phosphate. These precursors are dissolved in an appropriate solvent, such as ethanol or water, to form a homogeneous solution.

This method involves the conversion of a sol, a colloidal suspension of nanoparticles in a liquid medium, into a gel-like material through hydrolysis and condensation reactions. During hydrolysis, water molecules react with the precursor species, resulting in the formation of hydroxyl groups (OH^-) on the metal cations and phosphate anions. This hydrolysis reaction can be induced by adding water or a hydrolyzing agent, such as ammonium hydroxide or acetic acid, to the precursor solution. The hydrolyzed precursor solution undergoes condensation, where the hydroxyl groups on adjacent metal cations or phosphate anions react with each other to form chemical bonds. This process leads to the formation of a 3D network of interconnected particles within the sol, resulting in the gelation of the solution [6]. The condensation reaction can be influenced by controlling factors such as pH, temperature, and the presence of catalysts.

After gelation, the gel is subjected to an aging process, which involves allowing the gel to stand at a specific temperature for a defined period. The gel is then dried to remove the solvent and any remaining water molecules, resulting in a solid material. This can be achieved through various methods such as air-drying, freeze-drying, or supercritical fluid drying. The dried gel is subsequently calcined, which involves heating the material at elevated temperatures, leading to the formation of desired CaP product.

6.2.3 HYDROTHERMAL/SOLVOTHERMAL METHOD

The hydrothermal or solvothermal method involves the synthesis of CaP materials under high-pressure, high-temperature conditions in a liquid medium, such as water or ethanol. The precursor solution is typically acidic or alkaline depending on the desired pH of the reaction. The precursor solution is transferred to an autocalve, commonly made of stainless steel or teflon, capable of withstanding high-pressure conditions. The autoclave is sealed to maintain an airtight environment and prevent the escape of volatile species. It is then heated to the desired temperature, typically ranging from 100 to 250°C, and pressurized to high levels, often in the range of 50–200 atmospheres. Inside the autoclave, the precursor solution undergoes a reaction under the hydrothermal conditions. The dissolved calcium and phosphate species react and precipitate, resulting in the formation of CaP nanoparticles or crystals. Once the hydrothermal reaction is complete, the autoclave is allowed to cool down gradually to room temperature. This cooling step is essential to avoid rapid quenching, which can lead to undesired phase transformations or crystal defects. After cooling, the synthesized CaP material is isolated from the reaction mixture by filtration, centrifugation, or other separation techniques. The obtained CaP product may require washing to remove residual solvents or reactants. The isolated CaP material is typically dried at a moderate temperature to remove any remaining solvent. It can also further undergo calcination to remove any organic compound.

The hydrothermal/solvothermal method also allows for the incorporation of dopants or additives during the synthesis process [7]. By introducing specific ions or molecules into the precursor solution, researchers can modify the properties of the resulting CaP material, such as its biocompatibility, mechanical strength, or degradation rate.

6.2.4 ELECTROCHEMICAL DEPOSITION

Electrochemical deposition is a technique used to prepare CaP coatings or films on conductive substrates. The substrate is typically made of materials such as titanium, stainless steel, or other metals that have good electrical conductivity and are compatible with biological systems. The substrate is cleaned, polished, and pre-treated to ensure proper adhesion of the CaP coating. In this method, a conductive substrate acts as the cathode, and a calcium phosphate precursor solution serves as the electrolyte. The conductive substrate is immersed in the electrolyte solution, and a counter electrode, typically made of an inert material like platinum or graphite, is also immersed in the solution. The two electrodes are connected to an external power supply, creating an electrochemical cell. This counter electrode acts as an anode. Upon the application of an electric current, the calcium and phosphate ions from the electrolyte are deposited onto the substrate, resulting in the formation of a CaP coating. After the deposition, the CaP-coated substrate may undergo post-deposition treatments, such as rinsing with distilled water to remove any residual electrolyte or impurities [8].

6.3 VIBRATIONAL SPECTROSCOPIES

Vibrational spectroscopies play a vital role in the characterization of calcium phosphate (CaP) materials, providing valuable insights into their chemical composition, molecular structure, and bonding interactions. Mainly two types of vibrational spectroscopy- Raman and Fourier Transform Infrared (FTIR) spectroscopy are used to gain understanding of the composition, crystallinity, phase purity, molecular bonding, and spatial distribution of different CaP phases.

6.3.1 RAMAN SPECTROSCOPY

- **Principle:** Raman spectroscopy is based on the inelastic scattering of light. When a sample is illuminated with a monochromatic light source, such as a laser, a small fraction of the scattered light undergoes a shift in frequency.

This frequency shift, known as the Raman shift, corresponds to the vibrational modes of the sample's molecular bonds. The Raman scattered light contains information about the energy levels and vibrational transitions within the sample, providing insights into its molecular structure and chemical composition [9].

- **Instrumentation**- Raman spectroscopy utilizes an instrument called a Raman spectrometer, which consists of several key components: a laser light source, a sample holder, a monochromator or filter, and a detector. The laser light source emits monochromatic light at a specific wavelength, typically in the visible or near-infrared range. The light is focused onto the sample, and the scattered light is collected and filtered to separate it from the incident laser light. The filtered light is then dispersed using a monochromator or filter, and the resulting spectrum is detected by a detector, such as a charge-coupled device (CCD).

- **Advantages**

  1. **Molecular identification**- The Raman spectrum provides specific vibrational signatures corresponding to different chemical groups, such as phosphate (PO_4) groups, hydroxyl (OH) groups, and carbonate (CO_3) groups present in the CaP structure. This information enables the determination of the chemical composition and structural variations in CaP samples.
  2. **Phase analysis**- Different phases of CaP, exhibit distinct Raman spectral features, including peak positions and peak intensities. By analyzing the spectra, phase transformations and presence of impurities can also be detected. Raman spectroscopy can also be utilized to study heterogeneous CaP samples.
  3. **Non-destructive**- Raman spectroscopy is a non-destructive and non-invasive technique, meaning that it does not require sample alteration or preparation that could affect the integrity of the CaP material. The analysis can be performed on a variety of sample forms, including solids, liquids, and powders, without the need for extensive sample preparation.

- **Limitations**

  1. **Fluorescence**- Some CaP samples, particularly those containing organic components or impurities, may exhibit fluorescence, which can interfere with Raman measurements. Fluorescence can cause unwanted background signals that can obscure the Raman spectra. Strategies such as background subtraction can help mitigate this limitation.
  2. **Surface sensitivity**- Raman spectroscopy is generally more surface-sensitive compared to other techniques. It provides information primarily from the sample's surface, which may limit the analysis of bulk properties.

3. **Quantitative analysis**- The intensity of Raman bands does not always correlate linearly with the concentration or composition of specific components in the sample.

When performing Raman spectroscopy, the laser beam needs to be accurately focused on the sample for optimal results. If the laser light is precisely focused, it concentrates more energy on the sample, leading to a higher temperature increase within the material. Consequently, this elevated temperature causes the molecular bonds in the sample to vibrate more vigorously, resulting in wavenumber shifts in the Raman bands. Also, loosely compacted powders have more open spaces and less efficient heat dissipation, allowing them to absorb and retain more energy from the laser beam. As a result, they tend to reach higher temperatures compared to well-compacted powders, which have a denser structure and better heat dissipation properties. Precise laser focusing and denser sample compaction can minimize excessive heating effects, leading to more reliable and accurate Raman spectroscopic measurements [10].

6.3.2 FOURIER TRANSFORM INFRARED SPECTROSCOPY

- **Principle:** FTIR spectroscopy is based on the interaction of molecules with infrared radiation. Molecules can absorb infrared light at specific frequencies corresponding to the vibrational modes of their chemical bonds. When infrared light passes through a sample, it either gets transmitted, absorbed, or scattered. The transmitted light is measured, and the resulting spectrum, called an infrared spectrum or infrared absorption spectrum, provides information about the sample's molecular vibrations [11].

- **Instrumentation:** FTIR spectroscopy utilizes an instrument called an FTIR spectrometer, which consists of three main components: a source of infrared radiation, a sample holder, and a detector. The source emits a beam of infrared radiation, typically generated using a heated filament or a laser. The beam is directed toward the sample, which can be in different forms, such as a solid pellet, a liquid film, or a gas cell. The sample interacts with the infrared radiation, and the resulting transmitted or absorbed light is detected by the detector.

- **Advantages**

  1. **Chemical identification:** FTIR spectroscopy allows for the identification and characterization of different chemical groups and functional units within CaP materials. The absorption bands in the infrared spectrum provide specific information about the presence of phosphate (PO_4) groups, hydroxyl (OH) groups, and other functional groups within the CaP structure.

  2. **Phase analysis:** Different phases, such as hydroxyapatite (HAp) and tricalcium phosphate (TCP), exhibit distinct infrared absorption bands, allowing for the identification and quantification of different phases present in CaP samples.

3. **Structural analysis:** The shape and intensity of the infrared absorption bands provide insights into the molecular structure and bonding environment within CaP materials. Changes in the absorption band positions and intensities can indicate variations in the crystallinity.
4. **Non-destructive:** FTIR spectroscopy is a non-destructive technique, meaning that it does not require sample preparation that alters or damages the CaP material. The sample can be analyzed without any chemical treatment or modification, preserving its integrity for further characterization or use in applications.

- **Limitations**
  1. **Water absorption:** Water molecules strongly absorb infrared radiation in certain regions of the spectrum, limiting the analysis of CaP samples with significant water content. Special measures, such as sample dehydration or the use of specialized cells, may be necessary to mitigate this limitation [12].
  2. **Surface sensitivity:** FTIR spectroscopy typically provides information about the surface of the sample rather than its bulk properties. The depth of penetration of the infrared radiation depends on factors such as the sample thickness.
  3. **Quantitative analysis:** It may have limitations in precise quantitative analysis, such as determining the exact composition or concentration of different components in complex CaP mixtures.

Besides FTIR spectroscopy, XRD is also used for the characterization of hydroxyapatite. XRD helps in determining the crystal structure and morphology but does not comment on the amount or concentration of functional groups present in hydroxyapatite. Hence, FTIR is preferred more as it is a more sensitive technique and can detect small transformations in phase structure [13]. The maximum absorption peak in FTIR spectra is changed with a change in chemical composition of CaP. Small variations in the crystal structure alters the bonding interactions and hence, affects the frequency of the absorption peaks. By analyzing the peak width, one can assess the structural quality and crystallinity of the CaP material. A narrower peak suggests a higher degree of order and crystallinity, while a broader peak indicates a lower degree of order or the presence of structural defects.

6.4 RESULTS AND DISCUSSION

6.4.1 RAMAN SPECTROSCOPY ANALYSIS

Bertoluzza *et al.* observed Raman of tetra-calcium phosphate in crystalline form as shown in Figure 6.1(a). The lower vibrational modes (below 350 cm^{-1}) are due to the lattice vibrations. Some higher bands at 420, 567, 938, and 1017 cm^{-1} are observed due to the vibrations of phosphate ions. The highly dominated band at 938 cm^{-1} contributes to the symmentric stretching mode. Some lower intensity peaks lying between 983 and 1119 cm^{-1} are due to deformational stretching vibrations. Two

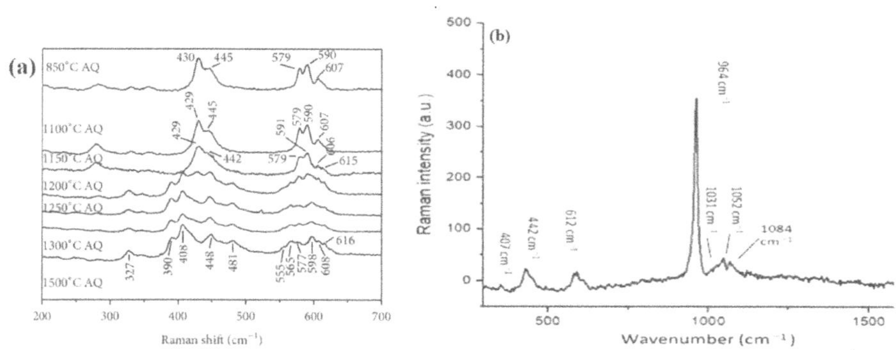

Figure 6.1 (a) Raman spectra of air quenched tetracalcium phosphate [15]. (b) Raman spectra of β-tricalcium phosphate [16].

medium intensity bands at 420 and 567 cm^{-1} can be seen both in infrared and Raman spectra. All of this data is coincident with the peak positions in infrared spectra [14]. Figure 6.1(b) depicts the Raman sepctra of β tricalcium phosphate. Raman spectra was recorded using an ISA U-lo00 Mole double monochromator Raman Spectrometer with resolution 4 cm^{-1}. The light source was a Argon ion laser with wavelength near to 488 nm and 100 mW power. The Raman spectra was recorded using the known raman bands of TiO_2 at 142 cm^{-1} [17]. Strong bands present at 938 and 970 cm^{-1} are due to symmetric stretching vibration of phosphate ions. Large prominent absorption band at 1048 cm^{-1} and a weak band at 1017 cm^{-1} is observed in both Raman and IR spectra of β tricalcium phosphate.

α tricalcium phosphate has 216 Raman active vibrational modes [18]. Two prominent bands at 964 and 976 cm^{-1} are present along with a weak band at 954 cm^{-1} as seen in Figure 6.2(a). Next, we discuss the Raman spectra of octacalcium

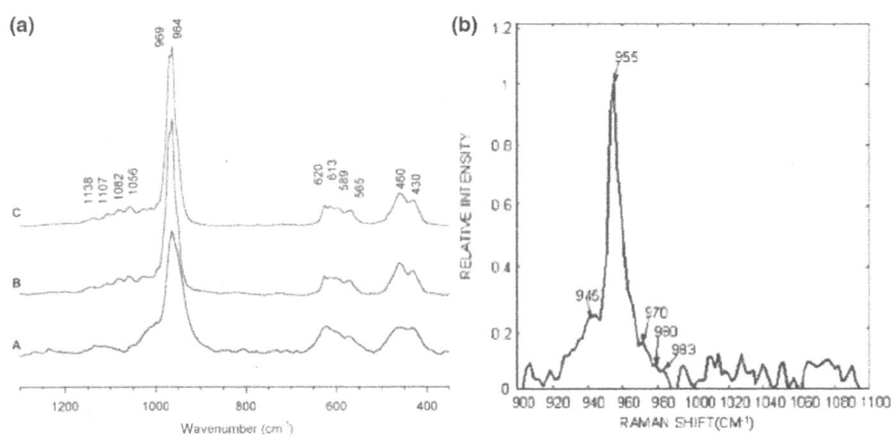

Figure 6.2 (a) Raman spectra of α-tricalcium phoshate [19], and (b) Raman spectra of octacalcium phoshate [19].

phosphate as shown in Figure 6.2(b). The bands at 916 and 879 cm^{-1} are due to stretching of P-OH linkage.

6.4.2 FTIR SPECTROSCOPY ANALYSIS

Figure 6.3 shows the FTIR spectrum of β tricalcium phosphate. Nicolet 60-SX spectrometer with resolution 4 cm^{-1} was used to obtain FTIR spectra. The spectrometer has a purging system to eliminate interference from water vapors and CO_2 in the environment. The infrared right was made to pass through the sample(in the form of pellets) and the resulting spectra was recorded.

Figure 6.4 gives a comparison between FTIR and XRD spectra of OCP. The spectrum of OCP has medium intensity peaks between 3000 and 3500 cm^{-1}. The

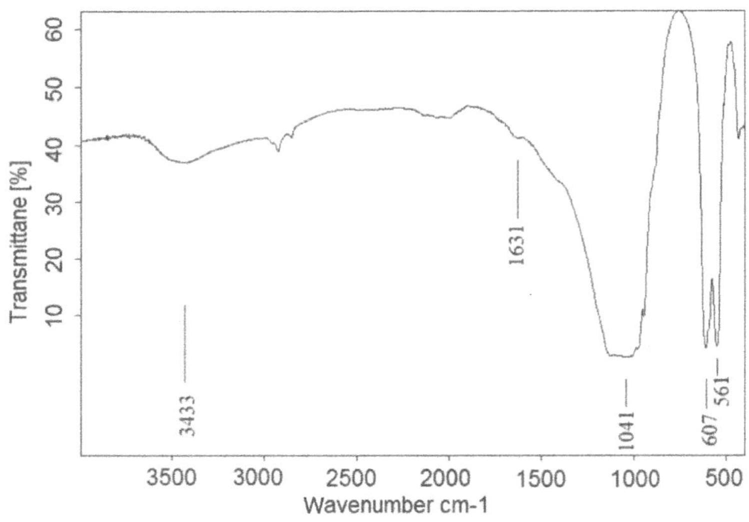

Figure 6.3 FTIR spectrum of β-tricalcium phosphate [20].

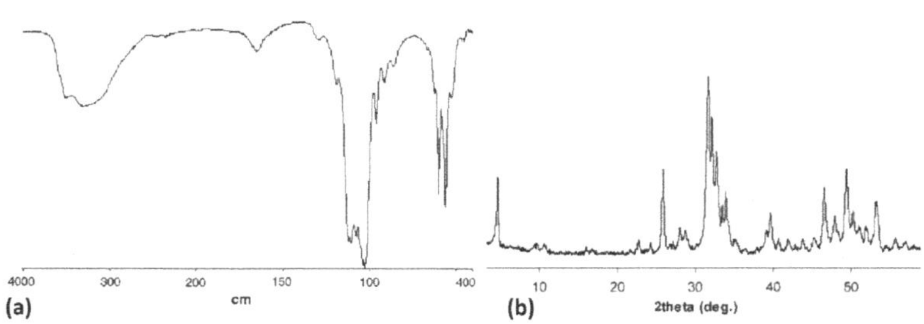

Figure 6.4 (a) FTIR spectrum. (b) XRD pattern of octacalcium phosphate [23].

peaks are slightly reduced after heating the sample to 100 °C. The peak at 1190 cm^{-1} due to stretching vibrations of phosphate ions gets shifted to 1240 cm^{-1} after heating. A weak band at 3565 cm^{-1} is observed after heating the sample to 150 °C. All the other peaks decreased in terms of intensity. Another minor band corresponding to the stretching vibrations of phosphorus to oxygen ions linkage was seen at 720 cm^{-1}. Peaks at 1280, 1240, and 910 cm^{-1} were not seen in IR spectra after heating OCP sample to 200 °C. Weak band at 1630 cm^{-1} remained till 400 °C due to the presence of water molecules in the sample. The IR spectra of OCP sample heated to 700 °C showed no characteristic band at 3570 cm^{-1} [21,22].

6.4.3 INFRARED SPECTROSCOPY ANALYSIS

In Figure 6.5(a), IR spectra of HAP, OCP, DCPA, and DCPD is shown separately along with a mixture of 25 percent HAP, OCP, DCPA, DCPD each. Some peaks at 630 and 3570 cm^{-1} corresponding to OH^- vibrations were seen in IR spectra of HAP but not in β TCP. Additionally, a peak corresponding to pyrophospate group was observed at 725 cm^{-1} [24].

Prominent doublet bands at 3548 and 3490, 3281 and 3163 cm^{-1}, a weak shoulder at 2950 and 2390 cm^{-1} and a sharp band around 1652 cm^{-1} can be observed for the case of DCPD. The two strong doublet bands arise due to the vibrations of

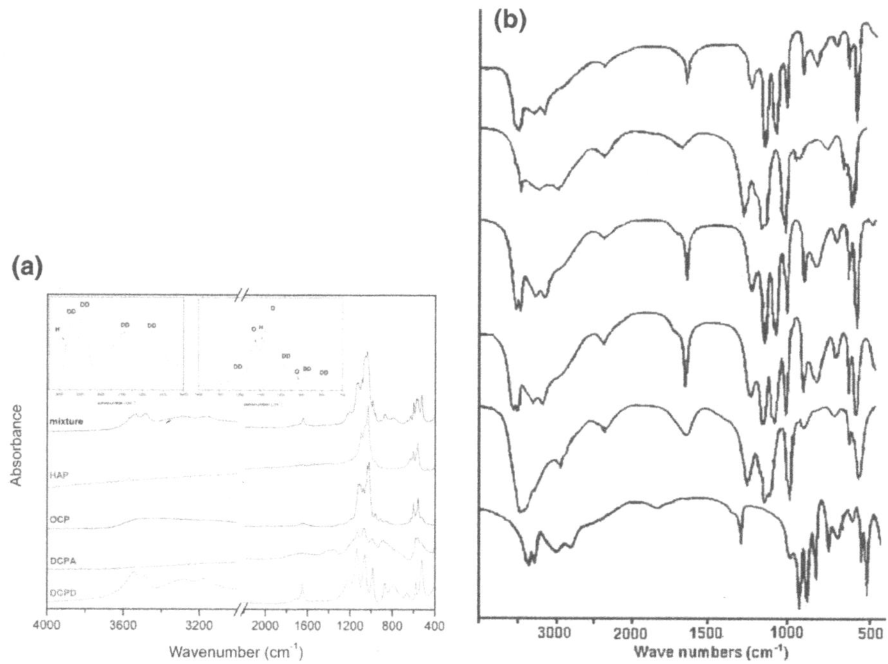

Figure 6.5 (a)Infrared spectra of different forms of calcium phosphate [11]. (b) Infrared spectra of monocalcium phosphate monohydrate [27].

water molecules and vanish when the sample is heated. The higher frequency doublet band is narrower and sharp while the lower frequency band is wider. The sharp intense band at 1652 cm^{-1} matches with the frequency of free water molecules and arises due to in-plane bending vibrations of water molecules present in the sample. For DCPA, peaks lying between 900 and 1200 cm^{-1} correspond to P-O stretching while the same band is seen at 988 cm^{-1} in the IR spectra of DCPD. The diffrence in frequencies is caused due to the stretching or lengthening of P-O bond. The band around 1217 cm^{-1} seen in DCPD spectra is due to the O-H in plane bending vibrations. The same broader band occurs below 900 cm^{-1} in DCPA spectra. A weak band at 790 cm^{-1} also appears in DCPA spectra at lower temperatures [25].

The IR active peak at 962 cm^{-1} observed both in HAP and OCP is due to symmetric stretching vibrations of phosphate ions. The bands at 865 and 910 cm^{-1} characteristic to orthophosphate vibrations help in identifying the mixture from OCP and HAP separately. A weak band at 525 cm^{-1} is only seen in OCP spectra and not HAP. Weak bands between 447 and 472 cm^{-1} may arise due to lattice vibrations [26].

Figure 6.5(b) depicts IR spectra of monocalcium phosphate monohydrate. Peaks at 3460, 3220, and 1650 cm^{-1} were observed corresponding to the asymmetric, symmetric and bending vibrations of water respectively. A weak absorption band is also observed between 1600 and 1700 cm^{-1}. However, IR spectra shows a strong large absorption band between 1000 and 1100 cm^{-1} which is not observed in its Raman spectra [28].

6.5 APPLICATIONS OF VIBRATIONAL SPECTROSCOPY IN CALCIUM PHOSPHATE RESEARCH

6.5.1 CHARACTERIZATION OF HYDROXYAPATITE [29]

- PO_4 *vibrations:* Phosphate (PO_4) groups in hydroxyapatite exhibit characteristic peaks in the FTIR spectrum, typically at around 960, 600–630, and 560 cm^{-1}. These bands correspond to symmetric stretching, bending, and asymmetric stretching modes of the phosphate groups, respectively. The symmetric mode is same in Raman spectra but bending and asymmetric peaks shift to 430 and 590 cm^{-1}, respectively.

- OH *vibrations:* Hydroxyl (OH) groups present in hydroxyapatite contribute to prominent absorption bands in the FTIR spectrum. The OH stretching modes are observed at approximately 3570 and 630 cm^{-1}. These bands provide insights into the structure and thermal stability of the hydroxyapatite material.

- CO_3 *vibrations:* In some cases, hydroxyapatite may contain carbonate (CO_3) ions due to biological or synthetic factors. The presence of CO_3 groups can be detected in the FTIR spectrum, typically with absorption bands at around 1460 and 870 cm^{-1}.

6.5.2 DETECTION OF IMPURITIES AND SUBSTITUTIONS

Vibrational spectroscopy facilitates the detection of impurities and substitutions within CaP materials. Subtle changes in absorption or scattering bands reveal the incorporation of foreign ions, such as magnesium (Mg^{2+}), strontium (Sr^{2+}), or fluoride (F^-), into the CaP lattice. This capability is crucial for tailoring the properties of CaP for specific biomedical applications, including drug delivery systems and tissue engineering scaffolds.

6.5.3 ASSESSMENT OF BIOACTIVITY AND DEGRADATION BEHAVIOR

The study of CaP bioactivity is fundamental for evaluating its potential in bone tissue engineering and regenerative medicine. Vibrational spectroscopy enables the monitoring of apatite formation on CaP surfaces during in vitro and in vivo experiments. Time-dependent changes in vibrational spectra reveal the rate of apatite mineralization and degradation behavior, providing insights into the material's long-term stability and interaction with biological environments [30].

6.5.4 CHARACTERIZATION OF COMPOSITE MATERIALS

Vibrational spectroscopy is particularly valuable for the characterization of CaP-based composite materials. By combining CaP with other biomaterials or bioactive substances, researchers can create tailored composite structures with enhanced mechanical and biological properties. FTIR and Raman spectra help identify the different components in the composite and assess their interactions, ultimately guiding the design of novel biomaterials for specific clinical applications.

6.5.5 QUALITY CONTROL

Vibrational spectroscopy techniques are well-suited for quality control and batch-to-batch consistency assessments in the biomedical and pharmaceutical industries. The rapid and non-destructive nature of FTIR and Raman spectroscopy enables real-time monitoring and validation of CaP materials used in medical devices, implants, and drug delivery systems, ensuring product safety and efficacy.

6.5.6 MONITORING OF CALCIUM PHOSPHATE COATINGS ON IMPLANTS

Raman spectroscopy, combined with suitable calibration methods, offers the capability to estimate the thickness of CaP coatings on implant surfaces. Raman spectroscopy measures the intensity of Raman scattering, which is directly related to the amount of material present in the probed volume. By comparing the Raman intensity to calibration standard of known thickness, the thickness of the CaP coating can be estimated non-destructively and in real-time. Monitoring changes in the crystallinity over time can help assess the stability and bioactivity of the coatings. FTIR spectroscopy can be employed to study the interfacial bonding between the CaP coating and the implant substrate. By analyzing the FTIR spectra at the interface, researchers can evaluate the presence of chemical interactions or any potential delamination issues, which are crucial for ensuring the long-term stability and performance of the coatings. Both FTIR and Raman spectroscopy offer the advantage of in-situ monitoring of coating degradation. Researchers can use these techniques to track changes in the vibrational spectra over time, providing valuable information on the chemical and structural stability of the coatings under simulated physiological conditions. This data is critical for assessing the long-term durability and biocompatibility of the coatings in vivo [31].

REFERENCES

1. J. C. Elliot. Structure and chemistry of the apatites and other calcium orthophosphates. *Studies in Inorganic Chemistry*, 1994.
2. U. Posset, E. Löcklin, R. Thull, and W. Kiefer. Vibrational spectroscopic study of tetracalcium phosphate in pure polycrystalline form and as a constituent of a self-setting bone cement. *Journal of Biomedical Materials Research*, **40**(4):640–645, 1998.
3. S. V. Dorozhkin. Calcium orthophosphates in nature, biology and medicine. *Materials*, **2**(2):399–498, 2009.
4. D. Shi. Introduction to biomaterials. *World Scientific*, 2005.
5. A. Yelten-Yilmaz and S. Yilmaz. Wet chemical precipitation synthesis of hydroxyapatite (HA) powders. *Ceramics International*, **44**(8):9703–9710, 2018.
6. K. Ishikawa, E. Garskaite, and A. Kareiva. Sol–gel synthesis of calcium phosphate based biomaterialsa review of environmentally benign, simple, and effective synthesis routes. *Journal of Sol-Gel Science and Technology*, **94**:551–572, 2020.
7. R. Karalkeviciene, E. Raudonyte-Svirbutaviciene, A. Zarkov, J.-C. Yang, A. I. Popov, and A. Kareiva. Solvothermal synthesis of calcium hydroxyapatite via hydrolysis of alpha-tricalcium phosphate in the presence of different organic additives. *Crystals*, **13**(2):265, 2023.
8. Z. Shao, J. Xia, Y. Zhang, H. Jiang, and G. Li. Preparation of calcium phosphate/chitosan membranes by electrochemical deposition technique. *Materials and Manufacturing Processes*, **31**(1):53–61, 2016.
9. J. A. Stammeier, B. Purgstaller, D. Hippler, V. Mavromatis, and M. Dietzel. In-situ raman spectroscopy of amorphous calcium phosphate to crystalline hydroxyapatite transformation. *MethodsX*, **5**:1241–1250, 2018.
10. B. O. Fowler, M. Markovic, and W. E. Brown. Octacalcium phosphate. 3. infrared and Raman vibrational spectra. *Chemistry of Materials*, **5**(10):1417–1423, 1993.
11. I. A. Karampas and C. G. Kontoyannis. Characterization of calcium phosphates mixtures. Vibrational *Spectroscopy*, **64**:126–133, 2013.
12. C. Rey, O. Marsan, C. Combes, C. Drouet, D. Grossin, and S. Sarda. Characterization of calcium phosphates using vibrational spectroscopies. *Advances in Calcium Phosphate Biomaterials*, 229–266, 2014.
13. T. Theophile. ed. *Infrared Spectroscopy: Materials Science, Engineering and Technology*. BoD–Books on Demand, 2012.
14. W. E. Brown and E. F. Epstein. Crystallography of tetracalcium phosphate. *Journal of Research of the National Bureau of Standards. Section A, Physics and Chemistry*, **69**(6):547, 1965.

15. J. Liao, X. Duan, Y. Li, C. Zheng, Z. Yang, A. Zhou, and D. Zou. Synthesis and mechanism of tetracalcium phosphate from nanocrystalline precursor. *Journal of Nanomaterials*, **2014**:186–186, 2014.
16. M. H. Al Refeai, E. M. Al Hamdan, S. Al-Saleh, A. S Alqahtani, M. Q. Al-Rifaiy, I. F. Alshiddi, I. Farooq, F. Vohra, and T. Abduljabbar. Application of β-tricalcium phosphate in adhesive dentin bonding. *Polymers*, **13**(17):2855, 2021.
17. A. Jillavenkatesa and R. A. Condrate Sr. The infrared and Raman spectra of β- and α-tricalcium phosphate [$Ca_3(PO_4)_2$]. *Spectroscopy Letters*, **31**(8):1619–1634, 1998.
18. M. Mathew, L. Schroeder, B. Dickens, and W. Brown. The crystal structure of α-$Ca_3(PO_4)_2$. *Acta Crystallographica Section B: Structural Crystallography and Crystal Chemistry*, **33**(5):1325–1333, 1977.
19. J. Kolmas, A. Kaflak, A. Zima, and A. Ślósarczyk. Alpha-tricalcium phosphate synthesized by two different routes: Structural and spectroscopic characterization. *Ceramics International*, **41**(4):5727–5733, 2015.
20. B. Mehdikhani and G. Hossein Borhani. Densification and mechanical behavior of β-tricalcium phosphate bioceramics. *International Letters of Chemistry, Physics and Astronomy*, **17**, 2014.
21. B. Fowler, E. Moreno, and W. Brown. Infra-red spectra of hydroxyapatite, octacalcium phosphate and pyrolysed octacalcium phosphate. *Archives of Oral Biology*, **11**(5):477–492, 1966.
22. E. Berry and C. Baddiel. Some assignments in the infra-red spectrum of octacalcium phosphate. *Spectrochimica Acta Part A: Molecular Spectroscopy*, **23**(6):1781–1792, 1967.
23. P. Habibovic, J. Li, C. M. v. d. Valk, G. Meijer, P. Layrolle, C. A. Van Blitterswijk, and K. De Groot. Biological performance of uncoated and octacalcium phosphate-coated Ti_6Al_4V. *Biomaterials*, **26**(1):23–36, 2005.
24. L. Berzina-Cimdina and N. Borodajenko. Research of calcium phosphates using fourier transform infrared spectroscopy. *Infrared Spectroscopy-Materials Science, Engineering and Technology*, **12**(7):251–263, 2012.
25. I. Petrov, B. Šoptrajanov, N. Fuson, and J. Lawson. Infra-red investigation of dicalcium phosphates. *Spectrochimica Acta Part A: Molecular Spectroscopy*, **23**(10):2637–2646, 1967.
26. A. C. Chapman and L. Thirlwell. Spectra of phosphorus compounds—i the infra-red spectra of orthophosphates. *Spectrochimica Acta*, **20**(6):937–947, 1964.
27. J. Sánchez-Enríquez and J. R.-Gasga. Obtaining [$Ca(H_2PO_4)_2 \cdot H_2O$], monocalcium phosphate monohydrate, via monetite from brushite by using sonication. *Ultrasonics Sonochemistry*, **20**(3):948–54, 2013.
28. A. Bertoluzza, M. A. Battaglia, Sergio Bonora, Patrizia Monti, and Rosa Simoni. Hydrogen bonds in calcium acid phosphates by infrared and raman spectra. *Journal of Molecular Structure*, **127**(1):35–45, 1985.
29. B. Cengiz, Y. Gokce, N. Yildiz, Z. Aktas, and A. Calimli. Synthesis and characterization of hydroxyapatite nanoparticles. *Colloids and Surfaces A: Physicochemical and Engineering Aspects*, **322**(1–3):29–33, 2008.
30. R. Ramakrishnaiah, G. U. Rehman, S. Basavarajappa, A. A. Al Khuraif, B. Durgesh, A. S. Khan, and I. ur Rehman. Applications of Raman spectroscopy in dentistry: Analysis of tooth structure. *Applied Spectroscopy Reviews*, **50**(4):332–350, 2015.
31. S. Shadanbaz and G. J. Dias. Calcium phosphate coatings on magnesium alloys for biomedical applications: A review. *Acta Biomaterialia*, **8**(1):20–30, 2012.

7 Nanocrystalline Calcium Phosphate-Based Biomaterials and Stem Cells in Orthopaedics

Sanjeev Gautam and Aarzoo Dhiman
Advanced Functional Materials Laboratory, Dr. S.S. Bhatnagar University Institute of Chemical Engineering and Technology, Panjab University, Chandigarh, India

7.1 INTRODUCTION

Biomaterials are compounds found in remedial or diagnostic systems that are brought into correspondence with tissue or bodily fluids but are not meals or medication [1]. Nanocrystalline calcium phosphate (CaP) based biomaterials have emerged as a significant area of research and innovation in the field of tissue engineering and regenerative medicine [1]. These materials are of great interest due to their unique properties, such as biocompatibility, bioactivity, and resemblance to the mineral phase of natural bone tissue. The synthesis methods for nanocrystalline CaP biomaterials encompass a range of techniques, including sol-gel, precipitation, hydrothermal, and biomimetic approaches, each offering distinct advantages and limitations in fabricating these materials with tailored properties [2]. Structural characteristics, including crystal size, surface area, porosity, and phase composition, play a crucial role in determining the bioactivity and biodegradability of nanocrystalline CaP, further enhancing its potential for tissue regeneration [3].

The exceptional properties of nanocrystalline CaP biomaterials contribute to their favorable biocompatibility, promoting the interaction and response of cells in the surrounding biological environment. The materials' osteoconductive and osteoconductive properties make them highly suitable for bone tissue engineering applications, where they can serve as scaffolds or coatings to promote bone regeneration and integration with host tissues [4]. Additionally, nanocrystalline CaP's ability to release biologically active ions, such as calcium and phosphate, can stimulate specific cellular responses and improve regenerative outcomes [2]. The broad biomedical applications of nanocrystalline CaP-based biomaterials have extended beyond

DOI: 10.1201/9781003360605-7

bone tissue engineering. These materials have found use in drug delivery systems, where they can act as carriers for therapeutic agents, providing controlled release and localized treatment. Furthermore, in dental applications, nanocrystalline CaP biomaterials have been utilized in dental composites, coatings, and fillers, enhancing their biocompatibility and durability [1]. Additionally, these biomaterials have been engineered into scaffolds to support soft tissue regeneration, such as cartilage, muscle, and vascular tissue. Nanocrystalline calcium phosphate-based biomaterials hold great promise in the realm of regenerative medicine and tissue engineering. Their unique properties, synthesis methods, structural characteristics, and broad biomedical applications make them valuable candidates for improving patient outcomes and enhancing the field of regenerative medicine [3]. Addressing the existing challenges and further advancing research will undoubtedly unlock the full potential of nanocrystalline CaP-based biomaterials, paving the way for innovative therapeutic approaches and transformative medical advancements.

7.1.1 SIGNIFICANCE OF STEM CELLS IN ORTHOPAEDICS

Stem cells are primitive biological entities that possess remarkable abilities for rapid proliferation, continuous self-renewal, seamless transition into specialized cell types, and the extraordinary capacity to rejuvenate and restore various tissues in the body [5]. These valuable sources can yield these cells: bone marrow, periosteum, adipose tissue, placenta, umbilical cord, blood, human amniotic fluid, dental pulp, synovial tissue, skin, and skeletal muscle. Stem cells possess unique characteristics, such as self-renewal and the ability to differentiate into specialized cell types, including bone, cartilage, and muscle cells. These properties make them a promising therapeutic tool in orthopaedics. Some other uses are shown in Figure 7.1. Among the plethora of stem cell types available, mesenchymal stem cells (MSCs) reign supreme in this context due to their widespread usage. Their versatility stems from their ability to be procured from diverse sources, including bone marrow, adipose tissue, and umbilical cord [5]. In orthopaedics, stem cell-based therapies have shown great potential in the treatment of non-healing fractures and bone defects. When introduced into the site of injury, stem cells can stimulate the formation of new bone tissue and accelerate the healing process. Similarly, in cases of cartilage defects and joint diseases like osteoarthritis, which result in the loss of cartilage cushioning, stem cells can aid in cartilage repair and regeneration. Mesenchymal stem cell (MSC) trials have shown their potential in addressing the most prevalent musculoskeletal conditions, with osteoarthritis being a primary focus. Osteoarthritis is a progressive joint disorder characterized by degeneration, inflammation, and discomfort. Despite extensive efforts, no truly efficacious remedy has been developed to fully restore joint structure and function. Existing treatments for osteoarthritis mainly revolve around managing symptoms and alleviating pain, rather than offering a definitive and lasting cure [4].

CARTISTEM, an innovative treatment using allogeneic umbilical cord blood-derived MSCs combined with a 4% hyaluronate hydrogel, has shown great promise in addressing knee cartilage defects caused by osteoarthritis. Approved by the

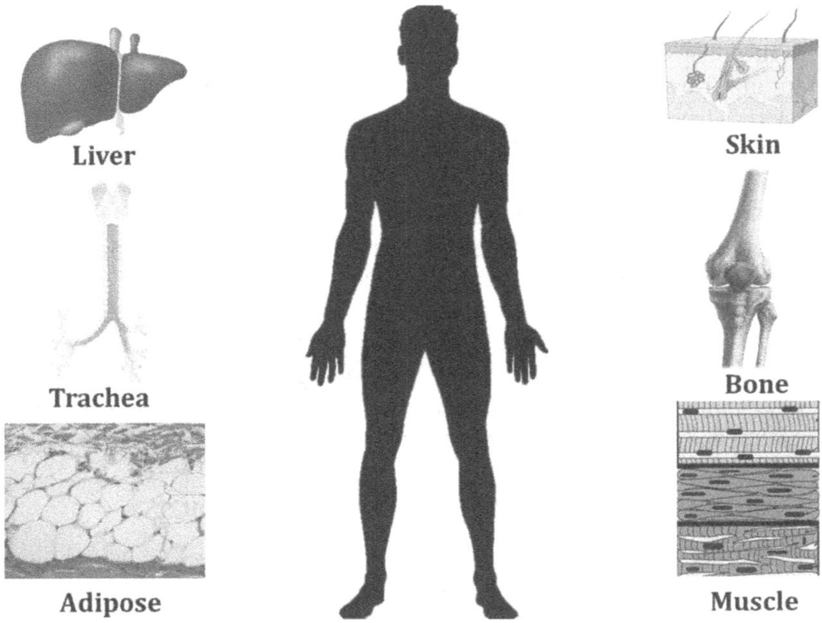

Figure 7.1 Illustration depicting area of biomedical applications of stem cell.

regulatory authority of the Republic of Korea in 2012, a clinical trial by Lim et al. in 2021 [3] found that 97.7% of CARTISTEM-treated participants showed significant improvement in cartilage repair compared to 71.7% in the microfracture group. These results highlight the potential of CARTISTEM therapy for restoring knee cartilage and advancing regenerative treatments in orthopedic medicine, offering hope for patients with joint disorders [3, 6, 7]

7.2 NANOCRYSTALLINE CAPO$_4$ BASED BIOMATERIALS

The human body relies on bone, a calcified substance, as a vital element to sustain and protect its functions. However, disruptions in bone integrity caused by factors like injuries, aging, infections, and tumors can profoundly affect an individual's health and ability to maintain a regular and active lifestyle. Nanocrystalline calcium phosphate-based biomaterials refer to a class of materials composed of nanoscale calcium phosphate crystals, which have garnered significant interest in the fields of tissue engineering and regenerative medicine [8]. One of the most prevalent types is nanocrystalline hydroxyapatite (nHA), which closely resembles the mineral component of natural bone tissue and is extensively used in bone tissue engineering, orthopaedic implants, and dental applications. Another type is nanocrystalline tricalcium phosphate (nTCP), valued for its higher a-solubility and faster biodegradability, making it suitable for drug delivery systems and as a temporary scaffold for bone regeneration [9]. Additionally, nanocrystalline amorphous calcium phosphate (nACP) stands out due to its unique amorphous structure, facilitating the controlled release of calcium and phosphate ions for enhanced osteoinductivity. Nanocrystalline biphasic calcium phosphate (BCP), composed of a mixture of nHA and nTCP, combines the benefits of both components, offering a versatile biomaterial for complex tissue regeneration strategies [10]. Table 7.1 has explained some of these types and their uses [11].

7.2.1 HYDROXYAPATITE (HAp)

Hydroxyapatite (HAp) is a highly researched biomaterial that closely mimics the chemical properties of the mineral found in bones. Among the various calcium phosphate (CaP) materials, hydroxyapatite (HAp) stands as the second most stable and insoluble, slightly falling short compared to fluorapatite (FAP). Its chemical formula is denoted as $Ca_5(PO_4)_3(OH)$. However, it is often symbolized as $Ca_{10}(PO_4)_6(OH)_2$ to emphasize the hexagonal unit cell structure of HAp [17]. Its crystal structure bears a strong resemblance to the natural hydroxyapatite found in bone tissue, contributing to its biocompatibility and facilitating the formation of a strong bond between the material and surrounding living tissues. This unique feature makes HAp a preferred choice for orthopaedic applications, where it plays a crucial role in bone tissue engineering, implants, and other surgical interventions [18]. HAp exhibits excellent osteoinductivity, providing an ideal substrate for bone cells to attach and grow, leading to enhanced bone regeneration and integration with the surrounding tissue. This property is particularly valuable in orthopaedics, where implants and scaffolds made from HAp can seamlessly promote new bone growth and restore damaged or diseased skeletal structures. Moreover, HAp's osteoinductive properties stimulate the differentiation of mesenchymal stem cells into osteoblasts, further promoting bone formation and healing processes.

In orthopaedic applications, the mechanical properties of biomaterials are of paramount importance. HAp possesses relatively high compressive strength and hardness, making it capable of withstanding the mechanical demands in load-bearing scenarios [9]. Although its tensile strength is lower than metals, the combination of HAp with other materials can lead to composite structures that balance mechanical strength with bioactivity, offering ideal solutions for orthopaedic implants and prosthetics. The biodegradability of HAp is another crucial aspect, particularly in orthopaedics, where temporary support is often needed during bone healing. Over time, HAp undergoes gradual resorption and is replaced by newly formed bone tissue. This property ensures that the implant or scaffold eventually integrates with the natural bone, avoiding long-term complications and enhancing patient recovery.

Furthermore, HAp's ability to release calcium and phosphate ions into the surrounding environment enhances its bioactivity. These ions facilitate cellular signaling and play essential roles in various biochemical processes, such as cell adhesion, proliferation, and differentiation. This feature is particularly beneficial in orthopaedic applications, where HAp can actively influence bone cell behavior and foster a conducive environment for tissue regeneration. Hydroxyapatite stands out as a remarkable biomaterial with characteristics closely resembling the mineral composition of

Table 7.1
Actual Term of Different Types of Calcium Phosphate

Type	Formula	Major Outcomes	References
HAP	$Ca_{10}(PO_4)_6(OH)_2$	The intervention focuses on stimulating M2 macrophages polarization, angiogenesis, and specifically increasing the production of IL-10, an essential anti-inflammatory cytokine with immunomodulatory effects.	[9]
α-TCP	α-$Ca_3(PO_4)_2$	The hydrothermal process holds potential for the microstructure with nano porosity and smaller nanopore size, leading to a substantial boost in bone formation.	[12]
β-TCP	β-$Ca_3(PO_4)_2$	The intervention specifically amplifies the expression of genes associated with osteoclast and extracelular space pathways, effectively promoting bone remodeling through enhanced differentiation.	[13]
ACP	$Ca_xH_y(PO_4)_z{\cdot}nH2O$	ALP incorporation in the biomimetic approach produces mineralized ACP nanoparticles enhancing BMSCs proliferation and osteogenic differentiation via ALP's bioactivity.	[14]
OCP	$Ca_8H_2(PO_4)_6{\cdot}5H_2O$	By promoting angiogenesis, the bone regeneration process is enhanced.	[15]
DCPA	$CaHPO_4$	The complete resorption of DCPA cement surpasses DCPD cement,with more substantial bone formation	
DCPD	$Ca_4(PO_4)_2O$	The intervention shows higher cell viability, ALP activity, and quantity, with reduced residual implant and remarkable new bone formation.	[16]

Abbreviations: α-TCP: α-Tricalcium Phosphate, β-TCP: β-Tricalcium Phosphate, ACP: Amorphous Phosphate Calcium, HAP: Hydroxyapatite bones. Its excellent biocompatibility, osteoinductivity, osteoinductivity, mechanical strength, and controlled biodegradability make it an ideal choice for various orthopedic applications. As researchers continue to explore and refine its properties, HAp is expected to remain at the forefront of orthopaedic advancements, revolutionizing the field of bone tissue engineering and improving the quality of life for countless individuals with skeletal disorders and injuries.

7.2.2 TRICALCIUM PHOSPHATE (TCP)

Tricalcium phosphate (TCP), being among the extensively researched calcium phosphate materials, exists in two distinct crystalline phases known as α-TCP and β-TCP. Several other phases of calcium phosphate materials share similar compositions with TCP. Here, the term TCP specifically refers to the phase with a chemical composition of $Ca_3(PO_4)_2$ and a Ca/P ratio of 1.5. Notably, pure crystalline α-TCP cannot be readily precipitated in aqueous solutions due to its extremely low solubility, in contrast to the more soluble β-TCP phase [19, 20]. One of the notable characteristics of TCP is its excellent biocompatibility, making it well-suited for medical applications. When TCP is implanted into the human body, it exhibits minimal adverse reactions with surrounding tissues, reducing the risk of inflammatory responses or rejection. This biocompatibility is a crucial feature, especially in orthopaedics, where materials must seamlessly integrate with bone tissue to promote successful bone healing and regeneration. TCP also possesses osteoinductivity, which refers to its ability to serve as a scaffold for bone cells to attach and grow. In orthopaedics, this property is vital for the development of bone graft substitutes and bone void fillers. TCP-based scaffolds provide a supportive framework for bone cells to proliferate and deposit new bone matrix, facilitating the natural healing process and eventual bone tissue restoration. TCP exhibits controlled biodegradability, particularly β-TCP, which gradually resorbs in the body over time, being replaced by newly formed bone tissue. TCP demonstrates outstanding stability and can be stored at room temperature in a dry environment for extended periods. A density functional study reveals that β-TCP exhibits greater stability compared to α-TCP [21].

The calcium and phosphate ions released during TCP degradation further contribute to its bioactivity. These ions play essential roles in cellular signaling and facilitate the recruitment and differentiation of bone-forming cells, promoting bone regeneration. TCP's ability to actively interact with the biological environment is particularly valuable in orthopedics, where it aids in enhancing the healing process and fostering a favorable environment for bone tissue growth. In orthopedics, TCP finds extensive use as bone graft substitutes, where it can be utilized alone or in combination with other materials to fill bone defects and promote bone regeneration. It is also employed in the production of resorbable screws and pins for orthopedic fixation, providing temporary support until the bone heals and then gradually resorbing to avoid the need for additional surgeries for implant removal. Moreover, TCP based coatings are applied to metallic implants to enhance their bioactivity and osseointegration, improving the long-term success of orthopaedic implants [21].

7.2.3 BIOCOMPATIBILITY AND BIOACTIVITY

Calcium phosphate exhibits remarkable biocompatibility, making it a highly coveted material in the realm of biomedicine. When in direct contact with living tissues, calcium phosphate materials provoke negligible adverse reactions or cytotoxicity [22, 23]. The biocompatibility of calcium phosphate-based biomaterials stands as a testament to their desirability and significance in the medical field. These biomaterials, composed primarily of calcium phosphate compounds, showcase a high degree of compatibility with living tissues, rendering them ideal candidates for various biomedical applications. Upon interaction with the biological environment, calcium phosphate-based biomaterials elicit minimal immunological responses, cytotoxic effects, or inflammatory reactions, underscoring their safety and effectiveness in medical interventions [24].

In a study conducted by Gao et al. [25], a calcium phosphate (CaP) material was synthesized and subsequently applied as a coating onto a magnesium alloy surface using a chemical conversion method. The biodegradation and biocompatibility properties of the CaP-coated magnesium alloy were compared to those of the uncoated Mg alloy. The findings demonstrated that the CaP coating exhibited superior cell behavior, proliferation, and adhesion compared to the uncoated magnesium alloy. Both in-vivo and in-vitro tests confirmed the enhanced biocompatible characteristics of the CaP-coated bio-implants. The study concluded that the application of the CaP coating significantly improves the biocompatibility of bio-implants, making it a promising approach to enhance the performance and acceptance of such medical devices in clinical applications [25].

The advantageous biocompatible nature of these materials facilitates seamless integration with surrounding tissues, fostering an environment conducive to tissue regeneration and healing processes. Their exceptional biocompatibility and harmonious interactions with the physiological milieu have propelled calcium phosphate-based biomaterials to the forefront of regenerative medicine and tissue engineering, offering promising solutions to address a myriad of medical challenges.

Calcium phosphate-based biomaterials possess remarkable bioactivity, making them valuable in various biomedical applications. They actively interact with the biological environment, promoting cellular responses and aiding tissue regeneration. Biomaterials like hydroxyapatite (HAp), tricalcium phosphate (TCP), and biphasic calcium phosphate (BCP) exhibit exceptional bioactivity due to their resemblance to natural bone tissue. When implanted, these biomaterials release essential ions like calcium and phosphate, stimulating cell adhesion, proliferation, and differentiation. Osteoinductive and osteoconductive properties of calcium phosphates play a crucial role in bone regeneration, prompting progenitor cells to differentiate into osteoblastic lineages [8]. Gradual resorption, replaced by newly formed bone tissue, further enhances their bioactivity, making them suitable for orthopedic applications and regenerative medicine. Surface characteristics like roughness, crystallinity, solubility, phase content, porosity, and surface energy significantly impact cell adhesion [8]. Overall, the innate bioactivity of these biomaterials holds immense promise in advancing medical treatments, promoting tissue growth, and improving patient outcomes in various clinical settings.

7.2.4 SYNTHETIC BONE GRAFT SUBSTITUTES

Synthetic bone grafts have emerged as valuable alternatives to traditional autografts and allografts in orthopaedic applications, addressing the need for effective bone regeneration and promoting improved patient outcomes. These grafts are biocompatible biomaterials designed to mimic the structure and composition of natural bone tissue, facilitating the regeneration of damaged or lost bone.

Nanostructured calcium phosphate cement (CPC) represents a class of self-setting synthetic bone graft materials that have garnered significant attention in the field of bone regeneration. The pioneering CPC formulation, developed in 1986, comprised a mixture of tetracalcium phosphate (TTCP: $Ca_4(PO_4)_2O$) and dicalcium phosphate anhydrous (DCPA: $CaHPO_4$) [26]. These innovative biomaterials offer remarkable potential for bone repair and regeneration due to their unique nanostructured properties, which enable them to set and harden in situ, conforming to the shape of the bone defect and facilitating effective tissue integration. The nanoscale features of CPCs contribute to enhanced cellular interactions and favorable bone responses, positioning them as promising candidates in the quest for advanced solutions in bone tissue engineering and regenerative medicine [27]. One commonly used synthetic bone graft material is hydroxyapatite (HAp), a calcium phosphate compound closely resembling the mineral phase of bone. HAp provides an ideal scaffold for bone cells to attach, proliferate, and deposit new bone matrix, promoting osteogenesis and facilitating bone healing [9]. Another widely utilized synthetic bone graft material is tricalcium phosphate (TCP), which comes in two crystalline phases, a-TCP and β-TCP. TCP demonstrates controlled biodegradability, gradually resorbing and being replaced by new bone tissue during the healing process. This property is particularly beneficial in orthopaedics, where temporary support is often required to stimulate bone regeneration [12]. Additionally, biphasic calcium phosphate (BCP) combines the advantages of both HAp and TCP, presenting a blend of osteoinductivity, biodegradability, and bioactivity, thereby offering enhanced bone regenerative potential [13].

Synthetic bone grafts can be combined with growth factors, proteins, or stem cells to further optimize their regenerative capabilities and tailor their properties to specific clinical needs. As research and technological advancements continue, synthetic bone grafts are poised to play a crucial role in revolutionizing orthopedic treatments, providing innovative solutions for bone defects, fractures, and other musculoskeletal conditions, ultimately enhancing patient outcomes and quality of life [5].

7.3 OSTEOINDUCTIVITY AND BONE INTEGRATION

Calcium phosphate (CaP)-based bio ceramics have gained significant prominence as the foremost choice among synthetic biomaterials employed for the reconstruction of damaged bone. These biomaterials, when implanted, undergo a gradual degradation process in conjunction with bone healing [22]. As a result, the implanted materials are gradually resorbed, while the bone tissue eventually regains its original geometry and functionality [28]. This natural interplay between the CaP-based bio ceramics and the bone healing process ensures an optimal integration and restoration of damaged bone, making them highly effective and widely utilized in various orthopaedic applications.

Osteoinductivity refers to the capacity of a biomaterial to serve as a scaffold or substrate for bone-forming cells, promoting their attachment, proliferation, and differentiation. This property is crucial in guiding and facilitating the formation of new bone tissue on the surface of the biomaterial [29]. On the other hand, bone integration refers to the seamless incorporation and bonding of the biomaterial with the surrounding host bone. Successful bone integration ensures mechanical stability, load-bearing capability, and long-term durability of orthopaedic implants or bone graft substitutes. Achieving optimal osteoinductivity and bone integration is paramount to the success of bone regenerative therapies, as it directly influences the healing process and ultimate functional restoration of damaged or diseased bone [30].

As shown in Figure 7.2 the healing process comprises three overlapping stages: inflammation, proliferation, and remodeling. In the inflammation phase, injured tissues trigger an immune response to remove damaged cells and debris, setting the groundwork for subsequent repair. The proliferation stage involves the migration and proliferation of new cells to the wound site, as well as the formation of a temporary scaffold of granulation tissue. During this phase, blood vessels and collagen are laid down to support tissue growth. Lastly, in the remodeling stage, the newly formed tissue undergoes restructuring and maturation, aligning along the lines of mechanical stress and optimizing its strength and functionality. These three interlinked stages collectively contribute to the comprehensive and orchestrated process of healing in the human body [25].

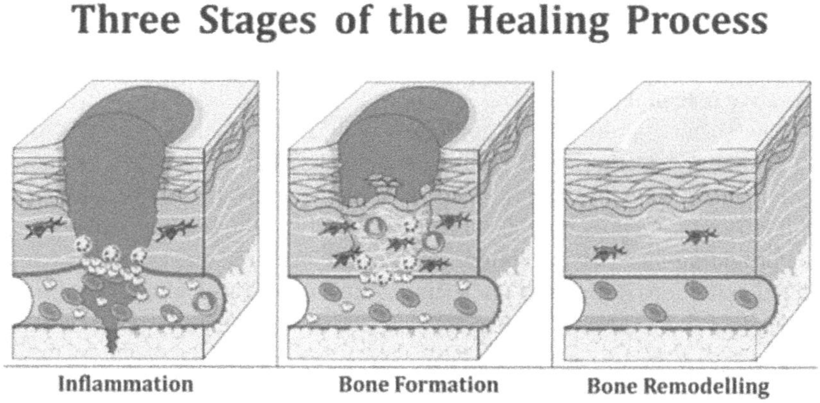

Figure 7.2 Illustrating the three stages of the healing process that overlap each other, namely inflammation, proliferation, and remodeling. These critical stages involve a complex interplay of cellular and molecular events, guiding the repair and regeneration of damaged tissues. (Adapted with permission under an open access CC BY licence from Gushiken *et al.* Life, 11:665, 2021. Copyright ©2021 MDPI.)

7.3.1 NANOCRYSTALLINE STRUCTURE AND ENHANCED OSTEOCONDUCTIVITY

One prominent benefit of nanocrystalline structures is their enhanced osteoconductivity, the ability to support the adhesion and growth of bone-forming cells. The increased surface area and fine-grained structure of nanocrystalline materials offer more sites for cell attachment, promoting cellular interactions and signaling crucial for bone tissue growth and regeneration [16]. The nanoscale features also facilitate improved protein adsorption and the release of bioactive ions, such as calcium and phosphate, further promoting bone cell proliferation and differentiation. The combination of nanocrystalline structure and enhanced osteoconductivity holds immense promise in developing advanced biomaterials for orthopedic applications, offering the potential for faster and more effective bone healing and integration with host tissues [31].

The utilization of nanostructured biomaterials in bone regeneration is influenced by the intricate architecture found in natural bone. Native bone possesses a sophisticated nanocomposite structure, primarily consisting of type I collagen in an organic phase, arranged as nanofibers with diameters ranging from 50 to 500 nm. Concurrently, the inorganic phase encompasses non-stoichiometric hydroxyapatite (HA) crystals, measuring approximately 100 nm in length, 20–30 nm in width, and 3–6 nm in thickness, expertly embedded within the collagen fibers. This well-organized nanoscale arrangement in bone serves as a model for developing advanced biomaterials that mimic the native bone structure, potentially enhancing the effectiveness of bone regeneration strategies and promoting better integration with the surrounding tissues [32].

CaP biomaterials replicate bone's inorganic element, exhibiting bioactivity and fostering strong bonds with adjacent bone, ideal for regeneration. Researchers explore various forms, like monocalcium phosphate, dicalcium phosphate, octacalcium phosphate, and tricalcium phosphate (TCP). Using different methods, nano-CaP crystals with diverse structures have been synthesized, showing superior properties to conventional CaPs due to their bone nanocrystal resemblance [31].

7.3.2 CAPO$_4$ IN CELL ATTACHMENT AND PROLIFERATION

Calcium phosphate biomaterials play a crucial role in tissue engineering and regenerative medicine, particularly for bone regeneration. Their biocompatibility and resemblance to natural bone tissue support cell attachment and proliferation [22]. The nanostructured topography and surface chemistry create favorable microenvironments that promote initial cell adhesion and interactions, laying the groundwork for tissue regeneration. The unique nanocrystalline structure enhances their utility as cell proliferation scaffolds, providing ample surface area for rapid and efficient cell growth. This nanoscale architecture optimizes their performance in supporting critical regenerative processes [33].

Prior research extensively examined how various stem cell types, including rat and different human mesenchymal stem cells (hBMSCs, hUCMSCs, hESC-MSCs, and hiPSC-MSCs), strongly attached to CPC scaffolds with apatite nanocrystals [34]. Scanning electron microscopy showed firm attachment through cytoplasmic extensions, fostering cell adhesion, migration, and vital cell-to-cell junctions. Nano-apatite surfaces effectively supported stem cell proliferation, indicating favorable interaction with the nanostructured biomaterial.

In another investigation, a nanofibrous scaffold containing gradients of amorphous calcium phosphate nanoparticles was developed using a two-spinnerette electrospinning technique. Notably, the gradient regions exhibited remarkable improvements in the adhesion and proliferation of MC3T3-E1 murine pre-osteoblasts. This outcome underscores the significance of higher nACP content in achieving a more favorable cell response. The study emphasizes the potential of tailoring nanostructures to guide and optimize cell behavior when interacting with nanostructured calcium phosphate biomaterials [35].

It can be said, the interactions between stem cells and nanostructured calcium phosphate biomaterials have been thoroughly investigated, demonstrating their profound ability to support cell adhesion, proliferation, and functionality. The adaptability of nanostructures in these biomaterials offers the opportunity to fine-tune cell responses and opens new avenues for designing advanced scaffolds that optimize tissue regeneration in various regenerative medicine applications.

7.3.3 IMPROVING BONE INTEGRATION WITH IMPLANTS

Following implantation, calcium phosphate-based biomaterials engage in intricate and tightly regulated interactions with the bone healing process. Various cells actively participate in mediating the degradation and resorption of these biomaterials, a crucial step that creates the necessary space for bone and vascular tissues to proliferate. The physicochemical attributes of these materials also play a vital role in modulating the behavior of cells and tissues, further enhancing the biomaterials' osteoinductive potential [28]. Such interplay between CaP-based biomaterials and the dynamic bone healing process underscores their significance as biocompatible and bioactive entities that actively contribute to successful tissue regeneration.

In one, his studies Wang et al. [36] studied calcium phosphate cement (CPC) scaffolds with varying Ca/P ratios and observed intriguing effects on osteoclastogenesis. A higher Ca/P ratio (1.67) in CPC led to slight phosphate ion release, enhancing osteoclast differentiation. These released ions facilitated increased binding between RANKL and RANK, reinforcing robust NF-B signaling. In a rat calvarial defect model, CPC with a high Ca/P ratio showed improved osteoclast-mediated bone healing. The topographical structure and crystallinity of calcium phosphate materials were identified as additional factors influencing osteoclast activities. Fine-tuning the composition and nanostructure of calcium phosphate-based biomaterials is essential for modulating osteoclastogenesis and optimizing bone healing outcomes [36].

The presence of different calcium phosphate (CaP) phases in implanted biomaterials significantly influences the interaction between osteoblasts and osteoclasts in vitro [37]. Studies revealed that low hydroxyapatite (HA) content in biphasic calcium phosphates (BCPs) (5% HA) led to increased expression of positive coupling factors, like sphingosine-kinase 1 (SPHK1) and collagen triple helix repeat containing 1 (Cthrc1), in cultured osteoclasts. Further investigations explored the impact of distinct chemical compositions and crystal structures of HA/monetite (OCP) or HA/β-tricalcium phosphate (TCP) disks on osteoclast formation and the crosstalk between osteoclasts and osteoblasts [20].

Both OCP and β-TCP facilitated the generation of multinucleated osteoclasts, with OCP promoting complement component 3a (C3a) expression, and β-TCP enhancing the expression of EphrinB2 (EfnB2) and Cthrc1 in osteoclasts. These secreted factors, in turn, stimulated osteoblast differentiation and function [15]. The chemical properties, particularly dissolution and precipitation around OCP and β-TCP crystals, were identified as potential factors contributing to the similar and distinct cellular responses observed in these CaP phases. These findings provide valuable insights into the complex interplay between the chemical composition and crystal structure of calcium phosphate phases, impacting osteoclast-osteoblast crosstalk, and have important implications for optimizing biomaterial designs in bone tissue engineering applications [35].

7.4 STEM CELL THERAPY IN ORTHOPAEDICS

Orthopedic diseases encompass a broad spectrum of medical conditions that affect the musculoskeletal system, which includes bones, joints, muscles, ligaments, tendons, and other connective tissues. These ailments can range from common issues like osteoarthritis and fractures to more complex conditions such as scoliosis, rheumatoid arthritis, and osteoporosis. Orthopedic diseases pose significant challenges to individuals' mobility, function, and overall quality of life [37].

Stem cells hold immense potential in revolutionizing musculoskeletal therapies, offering the possibility of treating and even curing various orthopaedic conditions. Over the past two decades, the field of orthopaedics has witnessed a surge in stem cell research, encompassing diverse stem cell types, including embryonic stem cells (ESCs), induced pluripotent stem cells (iPSCs), and adult stem cells sourced from different bodily sites. Each of these cell types presents distinct advantages and drawbacks concerning their translation into clinical applications [29]. ESCs and iPSCs possess true pluripotent properties but face complexities in controlling their differentiation, leading to regulatory challenges that may hinder their clinical adoption. In contrast, adult stem cells, commonly referred to as mesenchymal stem cells (MSCs), exhibit more limited differentiation potential but offer the advantage of ready availability, especially in autologous settings. The unique properties of adult stem cells vary depending on their tissue of origin, further contributing to the rich landscape of stem cell research and its profound impact on the future of orthopaedic treatments [38].

7.4.1 MESENCHYMAL STEM CELLS (MSCS)

MSCs represent a distinctive group of adult stem cells with exceptional characteristics and significant therapeutic promise. These versatile cells can be extracted from diverse sources like bone marrow, adipose tissue, and umbilical cord, ensuring their accessibility and suitability for medical treatments [39]. MSCs possess the ability to differentiate into several cell types, including bone, cartilage, and fat cells, making them attractive for tissue regeneration and repair. Beyond their differentiation capacity, MSCs exhibit immunomodulatory properties, which enable them to regulate immune responses and reduce inflammation.

It can be used in improving conditions of patients facing Osteoporosis as they have tendency to differentiate into osteoblast cells. Other than these numerous investigations have corroborated the therapeutic efficacy of mesenchymal stem cells (MSCs) in promoting cartilage repair, as evidenced by findings from both animal-based and clinical research. These studies collectively support the potential of MSC-based therapies in addressing cartilage-related issues, underscoring the significant advancements in regenerative medicine for enhancing cartilage healing and restoration as shown in Figure 7.3(a–d). Osteoarthritis (OA) stands as the prevailing chronic joint disorder, distinguished by the gradual deterioration of articular cartilage, degeneration of menisci and ligaments, thickening of subchondral bone, and the emergence of osteophytes as shown in Figure 7.3(c). It has no cure but recently MSCs have been used to repair cartilage tissue because of their ability to differentiate into different tissues, including cartilage tissue as part of treatment [40].

Intervertebral disc disease (IDD) manifests as debilitating back and neck pain [38]. This condition is characterized by an upsurge in proinflammatory cytokine release, heightened macrophage migration, and the onset of extracellular matrix degradation [41] as shown in Figure 7.3(b). IDD is marked by a crucial indication of dwindling viable and fully functional cells, gradually replaced by a substantial influx

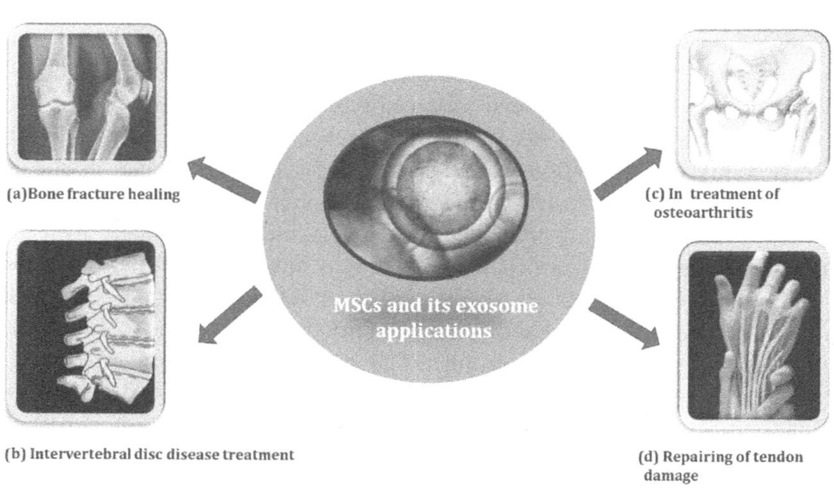

Figure 7.3 (a) The use mesenchymal stem cell exosomes in healing of bone fracture. (b) Mesenchymal stem cells and their exosome use in IID treatment. (c) MSCs for Osteoarthritis: chronic joint disorder. (d) Use of MSCs in repairing tendon damage due to their anti-inflammatory property.

of senescent and apoptotic cells. The application of stem cells has shown promising results in bolstering the viability of intervertebral disc cells, effectively impeding the progression of this debilitating disease [30]. MSCs is mostly used for its treatment as After transplantation, MSCs can differentiate into NP-like cells and stimulate proliferation in NPCs, leading to intervertebral disc regeneration [42]. MSCs exosomes play a pivotal role in regulating the inflammatory milieu, exerting a profound impact on nucleus pulposus cells (NPCs). This influence leads to heightened proliferation, reduced apoptosis, and enhanced extracellular matrix synthesis in these cells [43].

MSCs is also used in repairing tendon damage, as exosomes derived from MSCs exhibit remarkable anti-inflammatory properties by enhancing the migration of $CD163^{+}$ cells, representing anti-inflammatory macrophages, to the site of tendon regeneration as shown in Figure 7.3(d). Additionally, these MSC-derived exosomes possess the ability to influence macrophages, converting them into the M2 phenotype, which actively participates in anti-inflammatory and regenerative responses. This potent interplay between MSC-derived exosomes and immune cells offers promising therapeutic implications for promoting tissue repair and mitigating inflammation [44].

7.4.2 DIFFERENTIATION OF MSCS INTO OSTEOBLASTS

Osteoporosis is a common skeletal condition characterized by a reduction in bone density and strength, leading to a heightened vulnerability to fractures. This disorder occurs when bone resorption outpaces bone formation, causing bones to become weakened and prone to fractures, particularly in the spine, hips, and wrists. Osteoporosis predominantly affects older individuals, particularly postmenopausal women, due to hormonal changes that contribute to bone loss. However, it can also occur in men and younger individuals with certain risk factors [45]. The diagnosis and management of osteoporosis involve various approaches, including lifestyle modifications, dietary supplements, and medications aimed at preventing bone loss and reducing fracture risks [46]. This is mainly caused due to estrogen and glucocorticoid deficiency. Osteoporosis may result from disruptions in bone metabolic processes, characterized by an imbalance between osteoclasts, responsible for breaking down bone tissue, and osteoblasts, responsible for creating new bone. These disruptions can compromise the structural integrity of bones, leading to decreased bone density and increased susceptibility to fractures [47].

Research indicates that exosomes from MSCs show promise in boosting and protecting against osteoporosis. They enhance osteoblast survival, proliferation, and differentiation, especially in the hFOB 1.19 cell line, through the activation of the MAPK signaling pathway. The precise molecular mechanisms underlying this preventive action require further investigation [45]. MSC-derived exosomes contain essential GLUT3 protein and mRNA, crucial for osteoblast differentiation. Treatment of hFOB1.19 cells with these exosomes significantly increases GLUT3 expression, promoting robust osteoblastic differentiation. Additionally, exosome treatment upregulates pro-caspase 3 and 9 while reducing cleaved caspase 3 and 9 levels, indicating reduced apoptotic activity. This beneficial effect leads to increased cell proliferation and reduced apoptosis in hFOB1.19 cells, highlighting MSC-derived exosomes' potential as therapeutic agents for promoting osteoblast function and bone regeneration [48].

7.5 NANOCRYSTALLINE CAPO$_4$-BASED BIOMATERIALS AS SCAFFOLDS

Nanocrystalline calcium phosphate-based scaffolds exhibit the remarkable ability to release biologically active ions, such as calcium and phosphate, which in turn trigger specific cellular responses and foster tissue healing. Their inherent versatility and capacity to guide tissue growth and repair position them as highly promising contenders for developing advanced scaffolds in regenerative medicine. Notably, these biomaterials show particular potential in bone tissue engineering and other musculoskeletal treatments, showcasing their vital role in shaping the future of regenerative therapies and improving patient outcomes.

7.5.1 THREE-DIMENSIONAL SCAFFOLDS

Three-dimensional (3D) scaffolds are pivotal in tissue engineering, revolutionizing regenerative medicine. Mimicking the natural extracellular matrix (ECM) these frameworks promote cell attachment, proliferation, and differentiation. Designing 3D structures akin to native tissue fosters cell integration, yielding functional tissue constructs [12]. Furthermore, these scaffolds facilitate nutrient and oxygen diffusion, ensuring tissue viability. Versatile properties, including porosity, mechanical strength, and surface chemistry as shown in Figure 7.4, are tailored to specific tissue engineering needs. Material properties critically influence cellular behavior and

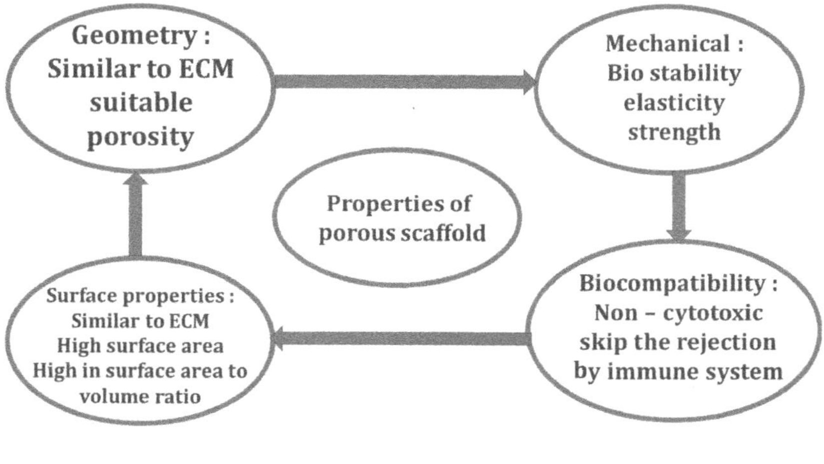

Figure 7.4 A critical view of various properties of porous scaffold.

fate, replicating the in vivo microenvironment. Scaffolds' mechanical and environmental cues drive tissue regeneration success. Precision in scaffold design remains paramount for achieving desired cellular responses and regenerating complex tissues in regenerative medicine.

In the realm of tissue engineering, natural polymers such as collagen, elastin, gelatin, silk fibroin, chitosan (CS), chitin, fibrin, and fibrinogen have gained widespread use in crafting 3D scaffolds, thanks to their exceptional biocompatibility [23]. Additionally, synthetic polymers like polylactic acid (PLA), polyglycolic acid, polyhydroxyalkanoate, and polylactic-co-glycolic acid (PLGA) have found application in scaffold preparation, owing to their adaptable porosity, degradation time, and mechanical properties as shown in Figure 7.5(a). In a 3D cell culture, these scaffolds act as the extracellular matrix, providing the necessary support for cells to maintain essential biophysical and biomechanical interactions. As a result, scaffold-based approaches present a promising avenue for advancing tissue regeneration and regenerative medicine applications [29].

Other than this, ceramics like tri-calcium phosphates (TCP) have been extensively employed in bone repair. The stoichiometry of TCP closely resembles the inorganic composition of bone, making it a preferred choice for bone regeneration applications. An outstanding advantage of α- and β-tricalcium phosphates lies in their water solubility, promoting enhanced in vivo degradation [22]. While αTCP is more soluble due to its specific crystallographic structure, it is derived from βTCP through high-temperature heating and rapid cooling. βTCP-based bone scaffolds typically feature porosity ranging from 35% to 50% and pore sizes spanning 100,300 μm.

Hydroxyapatite (HA), another widely used calcium orthophosphate compound, stands out for its stoichiometric resemblance to natural bone minerals. Various commercially available bone substitutes, including Pro Osteon 500R, Bio-Oss(c), and Endobon(c), are composed of HA. Pro Osteon 500R undergoes a conversion process from natural coral exoskeletons, leading to partially resorbable external HA and internal calcium carbonate. HA exhibits relatively low in vivo resorption rates at 5–15% per year [33].

Compared to βTCP, HA-based scaffolds exhibit a higher degree of crystallinity, providing mechanical strength akin to cancellous bone. Conversely, βTCP promotes degradation in vivo. To combine the benefits of both materials, composite scaffolds comprising βTCP and HA, referred to as biphasic calcium phosphates, are

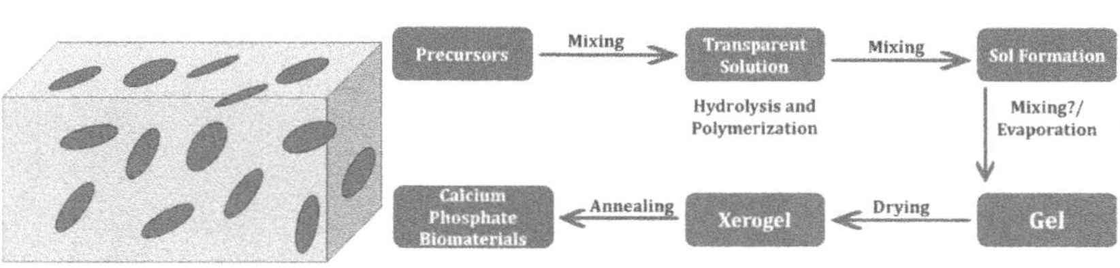

Figure 7.5 (a) 3D porous matrix type NCP scaffolds. (b) Sol-gel method for synthesis of NCP scaffolds.

employed. The resorption of these implants varies depending on the βTCP: HA composition, typically falling within the range of 40–60%. Prominent commercially available bone substitutes such as Triosite and BCP bone void filler embody these advantageous composite compositions [49].

7.5.2 SYNTHESIS AND FABRICATION TECHNIQUES

The synthesis and fabrication methods employed for nanocrystalline calcium phosphate-based scaffolds play a pivotal role in shaping their structural and functional characteristics. A diverse range of techniques has been developed to attain the desired properties of these scaffolds. One prevalent approach is the sol–gel method as shown in Figure 7.5(b), wherein calcium and phosphate precursors are blended in a solution and subjected to precisely controlled conditions, triggering the formation of nanocrystalline calcium phosphate particles [50]. Another technique involves precipitation, where calcium and phosphate ions are combined in an aqueous solution, giving rise to the formation of nanocrystals [49]. The hydrothermal and biomimetic methods entail specific temperature and pH conditions, closely emulating the natural mineralization process in bone tissue. These methodologies bestow meticulous control over the size, shape, and crystallinity of the nanocrystals [12]. Additionally, advanced fabrication techniques like 3D printing and electrospinning [27] have been harnessed to craft intricate scaffold structures, allowing for precise regulation of pore size, shape, and distribution. This adaptability empowers the customization of scaffold properties to precisely match the requirements of diverse tissue engineering applications.

7.5.3 CLINICAL APPLICATIONS

Within the field of orthopedics, nanocrystalline calcium phosphate-based scaffolds have garnered attention for their potential in facilitating bone healing and seamless integration with surrounding tissues. These scaffolds act as 3D structures, offering robust support for cell attachment, multiplication, and specialization, eventually culminating in the development of fully functional bone tissue. Moreover, these scaffolds provide a controlled release of biologically active ions,like calcium and phosphate, which prompt targeted cellular responses, thereby amplifying the regenerative results.

Moreover, nanocrystalline calcium phosphate-based scaffolds have demonstrated potential in dental applications, where they can be used as coatings, fillers, and bone void fillers in dental implantology. Their ability to support cell adhesion and proliferation in dental tissues facilitates effective integration with the surrounding oral tissues, promoting successful dental implant outcomes.

7.6 FUTURE PERSPECTIVE AND CONCLUSION

The continuous evolution of nanocrystalline calcium phosphate-based biomaterials necessitates focused research in refining fabrication techniques and exploring novel material combinations. Addressing critical challenges such as optimizing degradation rates and mechanical properties demands meticulous investigation and standardization of testing protocols. Interdisciplinary collaborations between materials scientists, biologists, and clinicians offer opportunities for personalized implant designs through advanced imaging and 3D printing techniques. Harnessing the potential of regenerative medicine, the incorporation of growth factors and stem cell therapies within these biomaterials holds promise for fostering more effective bone healing. Ultimately, nanocrystalline calcium phosphate-based biomaterials are poised to revolutionize orthopaedics, offering superior bone integration and regenerative capacity through innovative drug delivery systems and bioengineered constructs that mimic natural bone architecture.

In conclusion, the research on nanocrystalline calcium phosphate-based biomaterials for orthopaedic applications presents a promising frontier for revolutionizing bone repair and regeneration. The study highlighted the exceptional biocompatibility and bioactivity of these materials, making them ideal for cell attachment and proliferation, leading to improved bone integration with implants. To be specific mesenchymal stem cells (MSCs), are seen as significant players in orthopaedics, offering immense potential for differentiation into osteoblasts and synergizing with nanocrystalline biomaterials to enhance bone healing and functional tissue formation. Controlled drug delivery systems, featuring porous structures and localized release of growth factors, hold immense promise in promoting bone healing and boosting stem cell regenerative capacity. Integrating nanocrystalline biomaterials into 3D scaffolds offers an avenue to mimic natural bone architecture, paving the way for bioengineered constructs that revolutionize bone regeneration. As we look ahead, ongoing studies and interdisciplinary collaborations will drive the advancement of these innovative biomaterials, while addressing challenges in degradation control and mechanical properties. Standardized testing protocols will be essential for regulatory approval and broader acceptance. Embracing novel material combinations and continuous refinement of fabrication techniques, coupled with stem cell therapies, will unleash the full potential of these biomaterials, revolutionizing orthopaedic practices and instilling renewed hope in patients seeking bone repair and regeneration.

REFERENCES

1. T. Biswal, S. K. BadJena, and D Pradhan. Sustainable biomaterials and their applications: A short review. *Materials Today: Proceedings*, **30**:274–282, 2020.
2. S. Basu and B. Basu. Unravelling doped biphasic calcium phosphate: Synthesis to application. *ACS Applied Bio Materials*, **2**(12):5263–5297, 2019.
3. H.-C. Lim, Y.-B. Park, C.-W. Ha, B. J. Cole, B.-K. Lee, H.-J. Jeong, M.-K. Kim, S.-I. Bin, C.-H. Choi, C. H. Choi, J. D. Yoo. Allogeneic umbilical cord blood-derived mesenchymal stem cell implantation versus microfracture for large, full-thickness cartilage defects in older patients: A multicenter randomized clinical trial and extended 5-year clinical follow-up. *Orthopaedic Journal of Sports Medicine*, **9**(1):2325967120973052, 2021.

4. A. Mobasheri, G. Kalamegam, G. Musumeci, and M. E. Batt. Chondrocyte and mesenchymal stem cell-based therapies for cartilage repair in osteoarthritis and related orthopaedic conditions. *Maturitas*, **78**(3):188–198, 2014.
5. R. Mafi, S. Hindocha, P. Mafi, M. Griffin, and W. S. Khan. Sources of adult mesenchymal stem cells applicable for musculoskeletal applications—A systematic review of the literature. *The Open Orthopaedics Journal*, **5**:242, 2011.
6. D. K. Bae, K. H. Yoon, and S. J. Song. Cartilage healing after microfracture in osteoarthritic knees. *Arthroscopy: The Journal of Arthroscopic & Related Surgery*, **22**(4):367–374, 2006.
7. Y.-M. Yen, B. Cascio, L. O'Brien, S. Stalzer, P. J. Millett, and J. R. Steadman. Treatment of osteoarthritis of the knee with microfracture and rehabilitation. *Medicine & Science in Sports & Exercise*, **40**(2):200–205, 2008.
8. S. Samavedi, A. R. Whittington, and A. S. Goldstein. Calcium phosphate ceramics in bone tissue engineering: A review of properties and their influence on cell behavior. *Acta biomaterialia*, **9**(9):8037–8045, 2013.
9. O. R. Mahon, D. C. Browe, T. Gonzalez-Fernandez, P. Pitacco, I. T. Whelan, S. Von Euw, C. Hobbs, V. Nicolosi, K. T. Cunningham, K. H. G. Mills, D. J. Kelly. Nano-particle mediated M2 macrophage polarization enhances bone formation and MSC osteogenesis in an IL-10 dependent manner. *Biomaterials*, **239**:119833, 2020.
10. D. Xiao, J. Zhang, C. Zhang, D. Barbieri, H. Yuan, L. Moroni, and G. Feng. The role of calcium phosphate surface structure in osteogenesis and the mechanisms involved. *Acta biomaterialia*, **106**:22–33, 2020.
11. N. Eliaz and N. Metoki. Calcium phosphate bioceramics: A review of their history, structure, properties, coating technologies and biomedical applications. *Materials*, **10**(4):334, 2017.
12. Y. Raymond, M. Bonany, C. Lehmann, E. Thorel, R. Benítez, J. Franch, M. Espanol, X. Solé-Martí, M.-C. Manzanares, C. Canal, M. P. Ginebra. Hydrothermal processing of 3D-printed calcium phosphate scaffolds enhances bone formation in vivo: A comparison with biomimetic treatment. *Acta biomaterialia*, **135**:671–688, 2021.
13. C. Ji, M. Qiu, H. Ruan, C. Li, L. Cheng, J. Wang, C. Li, J. Qi, W. Cui, and L. Deng. Transcriptome analysis revealed the symbiosis niche of 3D scaffolds to accelerate bone defect healing. *Advanced Science*, **9**(8):2105194, 2022.
14. Z. Zhou, Y. Fan, Y. Jiang, S. Shi, C. Xue, X. Zhao, S. Tan, X. Chen, C. Feng, Y. Zhu, J. Yan. Mineralized enzyme-based biomaterials with superior bioactivities for bone regeneration. *ACS Applied Materials & Interfaces*, **14**(32):36315–36330, 2022.
15. T. Kurobane, Y. Shiwaku, T. Anada, R. Hamai, K. Tsuchiya, K. Baba, M. Iikubo, T. Takahashi, and O. Suzuki. Angiogenesis involvement by octacalcium phosphate-gelatin composite-driven bone regeneration in rat calvaria critical-sized defect. *Acta Biomaterialia*, **88**:514–526, 2019.
16. C.-L. Ko, J.-C. Chen, Y.-C. Tien, C.-C. Hung, J.-C. Wang, and W.-C. Chen. Osteoregenerative capacities of dicalcium phosphate-rich calcium phosphate bone cement. *Journal of Biomedical Materials Research Part A*, **103**(1):203–210, 2015.
17. B. Priyadarshini, M. Rama, Chetan, and U. Vijayalakshmi. Bioactive coating as a surface modification technique for biocompatible metallic implants: A review. *Journal of Asian Ceramic Societies*, **7**(4):397–406, 2019.
18. D. Bhatnagar, S. Gautam, H. Batra, and N. Goyal. Enhancement of fracture toughness in carbonate doped hydroxyapatite based nanocomposites: Rietveld analysis and

mechanical behaviour. *Journal of the Mechanical Behavior of Biomedical Materials*, **142**:105814, 2023.

19. H. Shao, J. He, T. Lin, Z. Zhang, Y. Zhang, and S. Liu. 3D gel-printing of hydroxyapatite scaffold for bone tissue engineering. *Ceramics International*, **45**(1):1163–1170, 2019.
20. M. Bohner, B. Le Gars Santoni, and N. Döbelin. β-tricalcium phosphate for bone substitution: Synthesis and properties. Acta Biomaterialia, **113**:23–41, 2020.
21. X. Guo, L. Lei, H. Xiao, and J. Zheng. Effect of remineralisation on the mechanical properties and tribological behaviour of human tooth dentine. *Biosurface and Biotribology*, **6**(3):92–95, 2020.
22. L. Le Guéhennec, D. Van Hede, E. Plougonven, G. Nolens, B. Verlée, M.-C. De Pauw, and F. Lambert. In vitro and in vivo biocompatibility of calcium-phosphate scaffolds three-dimensional printed by stereolithography for bone regeneration. *Journal of Biomedical Materials Research Part A*, **108**(3):412–425, 2020.
23. S. Mofakhami and E. Salahinejad. Biphasic calcium phosphate microspheres in biomedical applications. *Journal of Controlled Release*, **338**:527–536, 2021.
24. P. Dee, H. Y. You, S.-H. Teoh, and H. Le Ferrand. Bioinspired approaches to toughen calcium phosphate-based ceramics for bone repair. *Journal of the Mechanical Behavior of Biomedical Materials*, **112**:104078, 2020.
25. M. Maruyama, C. Rhee, T. Utsunomiya, N. Zhang, M. Ueno, Z. Yao, and S. B. Goodman. Modulation of the inflammatory response and bone healing. *Frontiers in Endocrinology*, **11**:386, 2020.
26. V. Karageorgiou and D. Kaplan. Porosity of 3D biomaterial scaffolds and osteogenesis. *Biomaterials*, **26**(27):5474–5491, 2005.
27. J. Zhang, W. Liu, V. Schnitzler, F. Tancret, and J.-M. Bouler. Calcium phosphate cements for bone substitution: Chemistry, handling and mechanical properties. *Acta Biomaterialia*, **10**(3):1035–1049, 2014.
28. Z.-S. Tao, X.-J. Wu, W.-S. Zhou, X.-J. Wu, W. Liao, M. Yang, H.-G. Xu, and L. Yang. Local administration of aspirin with β-tricalcium phosphate/poly-lactic-co-glycolic acid (β-TCP/PLGA) could enhance osteoporotic bone regeneration. *Journal of Bone and Mineral Metabolism*, **37**:1026–1035, 2019.
29. B. L. Seal, T. C. Otero, and A. J. M. S. Panitch. Polymeric biomaterials for tissue and organ regeneration. *Materials Science and Engineering: R: Reports*, **34**(4–5):147–230, 2001.
30. K. Lu, H. Y. Li, K. Yang, J. L. Wu, X. W. Cai, Y. Zhou, and C. Q. Li. Exosomes as potential alternatives to stem cell therapy for intervertebral disc degeneration: In-vitro study on exosomes in interaction of nucleus pulposus cells and bone marrow mesenchymal stem cells. *Stem cell Research & Therapy*, **8**:1–11, 2017.
31. Z. Xue, H. Zhang, A. Jin, J. Ye, L. Ren, J. Ao, W. Feng, and X. Lan. Correlation between degradation and compressive strength of an injectable macroporous calcium phosphate cement. *Journal of Alloys and Compounds*, **520**:220–225, 2012.
32. W. J. Landis and F. H. Silver. Mineral deposition in the extracellular matrices of vertebrate tissues: Identification of possible apatite nucleation sites on type I collagen. *Cells Tissues Organs*, **189**(1–4):20–24, 2008.
33. A. R. Vaccaro. The role of the osteoconductive scaffold in synthetic bone graft. *Orthopedics*, **25**:s571–s578, 2002.
34. J. Hernandez-Montelongo, D. Gallach, N. Naveas, V. Torres-Costa, A. Climent-Font, J. P. García-Ruiz, and M. Manso-Silvan. Calcium phosphate/porous silicon biocomposites prepared by cyclic deposition methods: Spin coating vs electrochemical activation. *Materials Science and Engineering: C*, **34**:245–251, 2014.

35. M. Ramalingam, M. F. Young, V. Thomas, L. Sun, L. C. Chow, C. K. Tison, K. Chatterjee, W. C. Miles, and C. G. Simon Jr. Nanofiber scaffold gradients for interfacial tissue engineering. *Journal of Biomaterials Applications*, **27**(6):695–705, 2013.
36. X. Wang, Y. Yu, L. Ji, Z. Geng, J. Wang, and C. Liu. Calcium phosphate-based materials regulate osteoclast-mediated osseointegration. *Bioactive Materials*, **6**(12):4517–4530, 2021.
37. J. Metzger and O. Distl. Genetics of equine orthopedic disease. *Veterinary Clinics: Equine Practice*, **36**(2):289–301, 2020.
38. P. Priyadarshani, Y. Li, and L. Yao. Advances in biological therapy for nucleus pulposus regeneration. *Osteoarthritis and Cartilage*, **24**(2):206–212, 2016.
39. C. Brown, C. McKee, S. Bakshi, K. Walker, E. Hakman, S. Halassy, D. Svinarich, R. Dodds, C. K. Govind, and G. Rasul Chaudhry. Mesenchymal stem cells: Cell therapy and regeneration potential. *Journal of Tissue Engineering and Regenerative Medicine*, **13**(9):1738–1755, 2019.
40. M. Kim, D. R. Steinberg, J. A. Burdick, and R. L. Mauck. Extracellular vesicles mediate improved functional outcomes in engineered cartilage produced from MSC/chondrocyte cocultures. *Proceedings of the National Academy of Sciences*, **116**(5):1569–1578, 2019.
41. J. Wang, Y. Tian, K. L. E. Phillips, N. Chiverton, G. Haddock, R. A. Bunning, A. K. Cross, I. M. Shapiro, C. L. Le Maitre, and M. V. Risbud. Tumor necrosis factor α- and interleukin-1β-dependent induction of CCL3 expression by nucleus pulposus cells promotes macrophage migration through CCR1. *Arthritis & Rheumatism*, **65**(3):832–842, 2013.
42. X. Cheng, G. Zhang, L. Zhang, Y. Hu, K. Zhang, X. Sun, C. Zhao, H. Li, Y. M. Li, and J. Zhao. Mesenchymal stem cells deliver exogenous miR-21 via exosomes to inhibit nucleus pulposus cell apoptosis and reduce intervertebral disc degeneration. *Journal of Cellular and Molecular Medicine*, **22**(1):261–276, 2018.
43. W.-R. Lan, S. Pan, H.-Y. Li, C. Sun, X. Chang, K. Lu, C.-Q. Jiang, R. Zuo, Y. Zhou, C.-Q. Li. Inhibition of the Notch1 pathway promotes the effects of nucleus pulposus cell-derived exosomes on the differentiation of mesenchymal stem cells into nucleus pulposus-like cells in rats. *Stem Cells International*, **2019**:8404168, 2019.
44. J. Wang, Y. Tian, K. L. E. Phillips, N. Chiverton, G.Haddock, R. A. Bunning, A. K. Cross, I. M. Shapiro, C. L. LeMaitre, and M. V. Risbud. TNF-α and IL-1β dependent induction of CCL3 expression by nucleus pulposus cells promotes macrophage migration through CCR1. *Arthritis and Rheumatism*, **65**(3):832–842, 2013.
45. P. Zhao, L. Xiao, J. Peng, Y.-Q. Qian, and C.-C. Huang. Exosomes derived from bone marrow mesenchymal stem cells improve osteoporosis through promoting osteoblast proliferation via MAPK pathway. *European Review for Medical & Pharmacological Sciences*, **22**(12), 2018.
46. Y. Ukon, T. Makino, J. Kodama, H. Tsukazaki, D. Tateiwa, H. Yoshikawa, and T. Kaito. Molecular-based treatment strategies for osteoporosis: A literature review. *International Journal of Molecular Sciences*, **20**(10):2557, 2019.
47. S. K. Sandhu and G. Hampson. The pathogenesis, diagnosis, investigation and management of osteoporosis. *Journal of Clinical Pathology*, **64**(12):1042–1050, 2011.
48. Y. Xie, J. H. Hu, H. Wu, Z. Z. Huang, H. W. Yan, and Z. Y. Shi. Bone marrow stem cells derived exosomes improve osteoporosis by promoting osteoblast proliferation and inhibiting cell apoptosis. *European Review for Medical and Pharmacological Sciences*, **23**(3):1214–1220, 2019.

49. N. N. F. N. Md. Noordin, N. Ahmad, M. Jaafar, B. H. Yahaya, A. R. Sulaiman, Z. A. A. Hamid. A review of bioceramics scaffolds for bone defects in different types of animal models: HA and β-TCP. *Biomedical Physics & Engineering Express*, **8**(5):052002, 2022.
50. O. M. V. M. Bueno, C. L. Herrera, C. A. Bertran, M. A. San-Miguel, and J. H. Lopes. An experimental and theoretical approach on stability towards hydrolysis of triethyl phosphate and its effects on the microstructure of sol-gel-derived bioactive silicate glass. *Materials Science and Engineering: C*, **120**:111759, 2021.

8 Zn- F-Co Substituted Nanocrystalline Hydroxyapatite for Bone Tissue Applications

Karishma Mahajan and Poonam Sharma
Department of Biotechnology and Bioinformatics,
Jaypee University of Information Technology, Waknaghat,
Solan, India

Vikrant Abbot
Chandigarh Pharmacy College, Chandigarh Group of Colleges,
Jhanjeri, Mohali, India

8.1 INTRODUCTION

Hydroxyapatite (HAp) is extensively used in bone tissue engineering because of its bioactivity and biocompatibility. Due to this, outlook of various researchers changes to explore new ideas for the further improvement in their physical and biological functions. Hydroxyapatite (HAp) is a significant calcium phosphate (CaP) compound that exists as a mineral phase within various natural hard tissues. It serves as an adhesive within the structure of natural hard tissues, playing a crucial role in determining the stiffness properties of bone, enamel, and dentin. The crystals within the collagen matrix of cortical bone are observed to be needle-shaped and aligned parallel to the direction of the fibres. HAp can be obtained from both synthetic and natural sources. Synthetic HAp with a stoichiometric composition of Ca/P = 1.67 has garnered significant attention in the field of hard tissue engineering. This is primarily due to its similarity to the mineral components found in the bones and teeth of mammals [1]. The least degradable form of CaP bioceramics exhibits exceptional bioactivity and biocompatibility [2]. HAp has strong chemical bonds with hard tissues because it is osteoconductive, doesn't harm the body, and doesn't cause an immune response [3, 4]. Consequently, HAp presents superior advantages in the realm of biomedical applications when compared to alternative materials used for bone substitution.

DOI: 10.1201/9781003360605-8

In the field of bone tissue engineering, there has been a lot of advancement over the last several decades in the search for a high-performance, low-failure, and long-lasting bone replacement material to use in place of auto-and allo-grafts in the treatment of orthopedic and dental abnormalities. Even with all the progress that has been made, finding the right biomaterial to aid in bone and tooth repair and regeneration is difficult. When organs are damaged or sick, doctors often turn to biomaterials to aid in the repair process. When compared to other bio-ceramics, pure HAp has the lowest biodegradability. According to research, HAp has osteo-inductive qualities and may speed up the bone regeneration process. When it comes to the management of bone infections, cancer, and other diseases, hydroxyapatite (HAp) possesses numerous significant applications as a bone substitute or replacement material in various contexts, such as, monitoring devices, bone or dental implant coatings, drug or gene delivery carriers, bone or dental fillers, imaging, complete or partial bone growth, and other related areas [5].

8.1.1 THE IMPACT OF IONIC SUBSTITUTIONS ON THE PROPERTIES OF HYDROXYAPATITE (HAp)

The use of pure HAp in bone-tissue engineering applications, particularly in load-bearing scenarios, is widely regarded as inadequate due to its inherent brittleness and lack of strength. Another big problem is the high level of crystallinity, which makes it harder for pure HAp to break down when it's in biological tissues. The presence of substituted ions affects the structure and composition of HAp Reports say that the biological response of pure HAp can be improved in certain environments by doping or substituting it with the right ions. The incorporation of precise elemental substitutions has been observed to modify the crystal structure, leading to enhanced biocompatibility and bioactivity [6]. This alteration has also been found to stimulate the responses of osteoclasts and osteoblasts, thereby contributing to the promotion of bone regeneration processes [7]. The incorporation of physiologically significant ions into the structure of HAp has been observed to have a beneficial impact on various physicochemical properties, including osteoconductivity, crystallinity, solubility, thermal stability lattice parameters, as well as enhancing its biocompatibility and bioactivity [8–11]. Furthermore, conducting research on ion substitutions in HAp holds significance and utility in enhancing our comprehension of the biomineralization process, crucial properties, augmentation of bioactivity, and its potential application as a drug carrier for the treatment of bone infections. Consequently, research on the synthesis of nanoscale HAp and its substitution with different ions has garnered significant attention in recent decades. Previous studies have shown that the incorporation of specific ions, such as cations (Mn^{2+}, Na^{+}, Sr^{2+}, K^{+}, Zn^{2+}, Mg^{2+}, or anions (Cl^{-}, F^{-}, HPO_4^{2-}, SiO_4^{4-}, or CO_3^{2-}), into the lattice structure of synthetic HAp can enhance its desirable properties [12]. The substitutions in question play a pivotal role in the biological activity that affects the morphology, structural size, solubility, and surface chemistry of HAp [13]. These substitutions elicit distinct biological responses in cellular systems [9]. The crystal structure of HAp exhibits the ability to incorporate substitutions of Ca^{2+}, PO_4^{3-}, and OH^- groups with diverse ions [14].

8.1.1.1 Zinc (Zn) Hydroxyapatite

Zinc (Zn) is a well-known constituent of natural apatite. According to reports, Zn promotes bone formation through osteoblast proliferation and biomineralization [15, 16]. It is involved in numerous enzyme reactions, including the replication of DNA and RNA and the synthesis of proteins. Zn aids in the metabolic processes responsible for normal bone growth and development, and its deficiency leads to a decrease in bone density [17]. Zn's biological efficacy is, however, dependent on its release behavior. The discharge of ions required for bone tissue regeneration should be regulated and gradual [18]. Due to the fact that the ionic radius of Zn (0.075 nm) is smaller than that of Ca (0.099 nm), it can be quantitatively substituted into the Ca (II) site of the HAp lattice by direct synthesis under moderate conditions. Its incorporation into the HAp lattice enhances thermal stability, modulates morphology, and promotes crystallinity [19]. The inclusion of Zn inhibits the growth of HAp crystals, and stoichiometry is no longer maintained, as the Ca/P ratio decreases as Zn mol% increases. Crystal strain has been reported to increase with increasing Zn concentrations, reducing crystallite size and crystallinity with increasing Zn content. The morphology of Zn-substituted HAp is irregular, with agglomerates growing in size as the amount of Zn increases [20]. Zn-substituted HAp particles exhibited high phase purity up to 800 °C, after which TCP began to form FTIR analysis revealed an increase in HPO_4^{3-} and a decrease in OH with increasing Zn concentration. Analysis of Zn-substituted HAp particles in simulated body fluid revealed the formation of a CaP layer at the particle's periphery. This biologically active layer strengthens the chemistry between HAp and bone [21].

8.1.1.1.1 The Significance of Zinc Ion in Biological Systems and Its Correlation with Calcium Phosphates

Zinc (Zn) is a trace element that is commonly observed in bone tissue. Human and animal metabolisms cannot function without it. In humans, its concentration in bone is between 0.012 and 0.0250 wt%. In addition to this, Zn contributes to the development and mineral formation of bone tissue. The growth of bones might be slowed down when Zn levels become excessively low [22, 23]. Zn has a stimulating impact on osteoblast cells and inhibits osteoclast bone resorption [24]. This is the primary motivation for Zn ion substitution inside the HAp lattice. Zn incorporation into HAp has been shown to reduce inflammatory cytokine production and boost anti-inflammatory cytokine production (by monocytes). According to certain studies, low-dose Zn supplements may boost bone tissue DNA and alkaline phosphatase (ALP) activity. Therefore, a Zn deficiency may slow bone formation. Diets low in Zn, ageing, and/or unloading the skeleton may all contribute to Zn loss. In humans, skeletal unloading increases the rate of Zn excretion during long durations of bed rest. Consequently, the appearance of extra Zn ions (after implantation) may encourage bone development surrounding the implant and also speed up growth of bone process in older adults. However, since Zn toxicity may occur at high concentrations, it is best to provide any extra Zn using a gradual release strategy [23]. When added to osteoblast cells, Zn stimulates their ALP activity. However, Zn deficiency has been linked to osteoporosis in the elderly due to its effect on the cell-mediated immune response [25]. Biological apatite is a calcium-deficient bone mineral with cationic or anionic substitutions. These substitutions improve synthetic HAp's properties, affecting osteoblast cell proliferation and osteo-integration over time [26–28]. Ionic substitutions into HAp are the subject of a substantial amount of study and development owing to the naturally high levels of zinc and other ions found in bone as well as the vital biological activities that are associated with them [28]. The ion-accepting HAp structure paves the way for the creation of novel, high-performance calcium phosphates with precise properties for a variety of purposes [29, 30]. Multiple ion substitutions have also been tried found that when Zn and F ions were co-substituted into HAp, cell proliferation and ALP activity were enhanced (along with mechanical qualities) [31].

8.1.1.2 Fluorine (F) Hydroxyapatite

Fluorine, in the form of F^-, is present in the skeletal structure and dental enamel of humans, serving as a vital element in preventing dissolution. Fluorine is a crucial element for the proper development of the skeletal system and teeth, as it is found in blood plasma and saliva. The substance is uniformly distributed within bone tissue and the outer layer of tooth enamel. The incorporation of fluoride ions F^-, into the HAp structure enhances bone tissue formation and subsequently enhances the response of osteoblasts in terms of adhesion, differentiation, and proliferation processes when compared to pure HAp. The process of substitution facilitates the establishment of a bond between bone and an implant, thereby enhancing the structural integrity of the bone [32]. Due to its low solubility, this substance effectively mitigates the process of bone demineralization. Additionally, it offers commendable acid resistance, a crucial attribute for dental health [33]. An optimal concentration of fluoride ions F^- facilitates the mineralization and crystallization of HAp during the process of bone formation. However, an excessive concentration of fluoride ions in bones can have detrimental effects, such as the development of osteomalacia [34]. The introduction of F ions into HAp results in favorable biocompatibility, reduced solubility, and enhanced thermal and chemical stability compared to unmodified HAp, as reported in reference [35]. Furthermore, the substitution of F ions has been observed to result in an augmentation of crystallinity, a reduction in crystallite size, and the introduction of crystal strains in hydroxyapatite (HAp) [36].

Fluorine, a vital trace element classified under the halogens group, plays a crucial role in maintaining human health by contributing to functions of nervous system regulation and the prevention of dental caries. In addition, fluorine has been found to have useful effects on the preservation of bone structure and functionality [37] Fluorine exhibits an affinity for a mitogenic stimulus that is conducive to osteoblasts, thereby facilitating the proliferation of osteoblasts and augmenting the process of bone formation [38] Moreover, scholarly research has provided insights into the preventive properties of fluorine in relation to osteoclastogenesis. This is achieved by inhibiting the development of osteoclasts and falling the levels of matrix tartrate-resistant acid phosphates and metalloproteinase 9 phosphates [39]. The application of fluoride to a titanium surface has the potential to enhance the production of osteoprotegerin, while also inhibiting activation and differentiation of osteoclasts. The synthesis of fluorohydroxyapatite (FHA) was achieved through the introduction of fluorine into hydroxyapatite. The goal of the study by Shibo Luie et al. was to find out if fluorine-modified hydroxyapatite (HAp) could still stop osteoclasts from doing their job in an in vitro setting. Therapeutic agents that can enhance the stability of implants in situations where osteoclast hyper function occurs Consequently, the study also examined the impact of these agents on the regulation of bone metabolism in an in vivo rat model of osteoporosis [40].

8.1.1.3 Cobalt Hydroxyapatite

Cobalt ions have been observed to induce a response similar to hypoxia and enhance the formation of new blood vessels and bone tissue, making them potentially valuable for applications in bone tissue engineering [41, 42]. A prior investigation demonstrated that the inclusion of cobalt ions within HAp resulted in an augmentation of osteogenesis in an in vivo setting. Although cobalt has been found to have beneficial osteoinductive properties, it is important to note that exposure to elevated concentrations of cobalt can have toxic effects on cells in laboratory settings and can also lead to pathologies in living organisms. The concentration-dependent effects of cobalt on osteoblastic activity were observed when the cells were exposed to cobalt in the culture medium [43]. Furthermore, it was observed that the leaching behavior of cobalt ions from the bioactive glass was contingent upon its cobalt concentration [44]. Hence, the identification of optimal cobalt content within Co-HAp scaffolds holds significant importance in the context of bone tissue engineering endeavors. In this current investigation, we conducted the synthesis and characterization of Co-HAp scaffolds with different concentrations of cobalt. Subsequently, we assessed the impact of cobalt on the degradation and bioactivity of the scaffold, as well as its compatibility with biological systems and the behavior and functionality of osteoblastic cells in an in vitro setting [45].

8.2 NANOCRYSTALLINE HYDROXYAPATITE

Nanocrystalline HAp powders have a more surface area, which makes them simple to sinter and densify. This could lead to improvements in fracture hardiness and other properties related to mechanical strength [46]. Furthermore, anticipated that nano-HAp will exhibit superior bioactivity in comparison to larger crystals. Therefore, the use of nano-HAp particles in engineered tissue implants can result in enhanced biocompatibility compared to alternative implants [47]. The application of nanotechnology holds promise for facilitating notable advancements in the development of HAp biomedical materials. In recent years, there have been numerous publications reviewing nanocrystalline calcium orthophosphates, as far as our current understanding goes. Dorozhkin et al. conducted a comprehensive analysis of the present technological advancements and recent progress in the field of nano-sized and nano crystalline calcium orthophosphates [48,49]. The research conducted in this study involved the production and evaluation of these materials, along with an examination of their potential applications in the biomedical and clinical fields. Tetracalcium phosphate (TCP) is used in a wide range of biomaterials, such as cements, sintered ceramics, and metal implant coatings. Moseke et al. did a full analysis of how it is made and what its properties are [46]. The investigation of calcium phosphate (CaP) and its polymer composites have been undertaken in order to explore their potential applications in bone regeneration and repair [50]. According to a summary provided by Tran et al., improved osteoblast functions have been demonstrated in nanostructured materials such as ceramics, metals, polymers, and composite materials. These findings were obtained in vitro as well as in vivo. These advantages include improved adhesion and proliferation, as well as the production of bone-related proteins and the deposition of calcium-containing substances [47]. We proceed to analyze its attributes within the context of nano-HAp which exhibits diverse morphologies and porous structures. These materials hold significant potential as viable alternatives for bone substitution and/or replacement in the realm of biomedical applications. This particular field of study has garnered significant attention in recent research endeavors [51].

8.3 METHOD FOR PREPARATION OF HYDROXYAPATITE

Numerous techniques have been devised to generate HAp with meticulous regulation of its structural characteristics. Sadat-Shojai et al. classified processes into dry, wet, high-temperature, biogenic synthesis, and combination categories. While solid-state and mechanical methods are examples of dry processes, chemical precipitation, hydrolysis, sol-gel, hydrothermal, emulsion, and sonochemical processes are examples of wet procedures (Figure 8.1). Sadat-Shojai et al. provide a comprehensive analysis of the synthetic pathways and properties of the resulting products, encompassing both scientific and economic aspects [52].

Method for the Preparation of Hydroxyapatite				
Dry method	*Wet method*	*High temperature process*	*Synthesis from biogenic source*	*Combination procedure*

Figure 8.1 Depicts graphical representations illustrating the various methodologies employed in the synthesis of hydroxyapatite.

8.3.1 SOL-GEL METHOD

The sol–gel approach is often used to produce metal oxides, ceramics, and glasses. The reactants are added in suitable solvents, leading to the production of a gel. The gel undergoes subsequent processing to yield the ultimate product. The sol-gel method consists of a sequence of discrete steps. Initially, the preparation of stable solutions of precursors is undertaken. Subsequently, polyesterification or polycondensation promotes the bridging of oxides or alcohols, which is the process by which these substances form gel. The third phase involves the solidification of the gel. Ageing is another term for this phenomenon. Dehydration and heat treatment are performed after ageing [53]. Calcium nitrate tetrahydrate is commonly used as main source of calcium. Diammonium hydrogen phosphate, triethyl phosphate ($(C_2H_5O)_3PO$), and phosphorus pentoxide (P_2O_5) are all examples of ionic sources for phosphate. As previously mentioned, the aforementioned solutions are combined to form a gel, which is subsequently subjected to a drying process prior to undergoing heat treatment. This heat treatment is typically conducted at temperatures ranging from 900 to 1250°C for duration of 1–15 hours [54–57].

8.3.2 CO-PRECIPITATION TECHNIQUE

Co-precipitation is the method by which particles form from precursor solutions while simultaneously nucleating, growing, coarsening, and/or agglomerating. The products resulting from precipitation reactions are typically composed of species that possess relatively low solubility and are formed when the solution becomes highly supersaturated. Nucleation is the main and crucial step in co-precipitation; it results in a large number of particles being produced. Following the nucleation stage, subsequent processes such as Ostwald ripening and aggregation are initiated. The size and shape of precipitates are controlled by processes that occur after the initial event. Typically, in order to achieve a stoichiometric ratio of HAp, the precursors are co-precipitated through introduction of basic solution, facilitating appropriate ageing [53]. A commonly employed procedure entails the incremental introduction of calcium, phosphorous, and Zc-containing precursors into one another, leading to prompt precipitation. Zinc nitrate is widely used as a prominent source of zinc ions. The addition rates of reactants typically exhibit a range of 5–30 ml/min. The pH is frequently elevated to a value greater than ten through the introduction of a base, such as ammonium hydroxide and sodium hydroxide. This procedure is implemented in order to guarantee the attainment of an apatitic phase in the final outcome. The ageing stage that ensues after the addition process may or may not involve the application of heat. The duration of ageing can typically range from a few hours to several days. The use of heat diminishes the necessity for extended periods of ageing. Following the ageing process, a washing procedure is employed to eliminate any unreacted precursors, if present, prior to oven drying. The oven drying is typically conducted within temperature range of 60–140°C, and the duration can extend up to 24 hours. Subsequently, heat treatments are commonly employed within the temperature range of 900–1200°C for duration of 1–15 hours in order to enhance the crystalline structure [58–62].

8.3.3 HYDROTHERMAL METHOD

The hydrothermal method, a process that involves multiple steps, entails a chemical reaction in which the solvent's temperature is elevated above its boiling point under significant pressure within a hermetically sealed container composed of either metal or teflon. In a batch hydrothermal reaction, ceramic sols are generally produced by chemical reactions that take place in the presence of an alkali or an acid under conditions of pressure and heat [63]. This pathway provides a sustainable and temperature based method for producing nano-sized particles, eliminating requirement for additional heat treatment. Undoubtedly, there has been a notable surge in the documentation of nanoparticle synthesis through the utilization of this hydrothermal method in recent times. As a consequence, immediate precipitation occurs. The composition, morphology, and crystallinity of particles are influenced by various factors, including pressure, temperature, pH, and ageing time. In contrast to alternative techniques, batch hydrothermal synthesis demonstrates the capability to generate single-step, crystalline, and phase-pure zinc-hydroxyapetite. The duration of ageing or vessel heating times can range from maximum of 24 hours. The reported synthesis temperatures in the literature exhibit a range spanning from 90 to 200°C. Furthermore, a limited number of researchers have documented the outcomes of posthydrothermal synthesis heat treatments conducted within the temperature range of 400–800°C for duration of 1–4 hours [59,64–66].

8.3.4 SOLID-STATE METHOD

The solid-state methodology is employed to synthesize Zn-HAp through the application of external force to induce a reaction between calcium, solid zinc, and phosphate precursors. Zinc-hydroxyapatite (Zn-HAp) was produced by Hattori et al. through the utilization of calcium hydrogen phosphate, calcium oxide, and zinc oxide powder. The powders were combined in purified deionized water and subjected to mixing in a ball mill. The mixed powder samples were subjected to heating at temperatures of 400 and 800 degrees celsius [67]. According to the findings of Hattori et al. [67], the authors reached the conclusion that the individual characteristics of the precursors were no longer discernible and instead an amorphous apatitic phase was achieved after a grinding period of 2.5 hours [68–70].

8.4 NANO-HYDROXYAPATITE AS A DELIVERY SYSTEM FOR VARIOUS CATEGORIES OF DISEASES

Nanotechnology refers to the theoretical and practical modification of matter within the range of approximately 1–100 nanometers in size. Nanotechnology plays a significant role in the exploration of distinctive and emerging phenomena as well as in the development of innovative applications. In the past decade, clinicians have been drawn to the study of engineered nanoparticles due to their various properties, making them a significant category of novel materials. Biomineralization and biomaterials both greatly benefit from the presence of nanocrystalline calcium phosphate apatite [71].

Kanaya et al. conducted a study in which they observed that n-HAp (nanohydroxyapatite) has capability of producing periodontal ligament (PDL) cell differentiation [72]. Mechanosensitive signaling and BMP-2 expression increase was revealed to be important for this differentiation. Additionally, Yang et al. found, in an animal research, that n-HAp has promise as a coating material on silk scaffolds [73]. Therefore, the researchers indicated that silk scaffolds coated with n-HAp have the potential to serve as promising biomaterials for the regeneration of periodontal tissue. In addition to the aforementioned studies, the extant literature contains several research articles that highlight the effects of n-HAp on various cells within the periodontium.

8.4.1 FIBROBLAST

Saleh et al. has been demonstrated that the utilization of silver nano-hydroxyapetite can effectively augment the maturation and proliferation of fibroblast cells. This has the potential to ultimately lead to the regeneration of connective tissue. In a study conducted by Shahoon et al., the biocompatibility of silver nanomaterials and n-HAp was evaluated on fibroblast cells. The results exposed that n-HAp exhibited significantly higher biocompatibility compared to silver nonmaterial's. It was discovered by Sun et al. that, in comparison to dense hydroxyapatite, n-HAp shown a better potential to promote the proliferation and differentiation of PDL fibroblast cells. Furthermore, it was noted that n-HAp exhibited higher biocompatibility compared to dense HAp [74, 75].

8.4.2 OSTEOBLAST

According to the research conducted by Shnettler et al., it was observed that n-HAp has the ability to adhere to the bone and activate osteoblasts during the initial phase of periodontal defect restoration [76]. This phenomenon has the potential to stimulate the process of osteogenesis. Thian and colleagues reported comparable findings in their study [77]. Furthermore, Pilloni et al. have demonstrated that the utilization of n-HAp has the potential to enhance the proliferation and differentiation of osteoblasts [78]. Webster et al. demonstrated enhanced protein adsorption and increased adhesion of osteoblastic cells to n-HAp in their report [79]. Liu et al. was observed that n-HAp had the ability to induce the adhesion and proliferation of osteoblast (MG-63 cells) [80]. Motskin et al. demonstrated the biocompatibility of n-HAp and its limited toxicity in osteoblast cells [81].

8.4.3 OSTEOCLAST

The research conducted by Detsch et al. demonstrated that the presence of low or negligible levels of carbonate in n-HAp can effectively promote the differentiation of cells like osteoclast. This phenomenon is able to lead to a higher abundance of osteoclast cells in the material in comparison to the carbonate-rich group. The activation of osteoclasts leads to the enrollment of mesenchymal cells from the bone marrow, which subsequently undergoes differentiation into osteoblasts. Furthermore, Matesanz et al. indicated that the differentiation of osteoclastic cells can be restricted by presence of n-HAp with silicon. As a result, a limited amount of bone resorption was identified on the surface of these cells [82, 83].

8.5 THE VITALITY OF NANO-HYDROXYAPATITE IN THE BIOMEDICAL FIELD

Nanoscale hydroxyapatite (nHAp) is getting a lot of attention in modern biomedical research because it has better surface properties than its microscale and bulk counterparts [84]. In addition to bioactive glass ceramics, nanostructured hydroxyapatite (nHAp) has been utilized in various applications, including coatings of dental implant, drug delivery systems, bioimaging techniques, processes of water decontamination, and technique for treatment of soil. Due to its significant contributions in the field of biomedicine, particularly in bone tissue engineering (BTE) and osteogenesis, numerous researchers have conducted extensive investigations on nHAp [85–91]. The enhanced sinterability and improved densification of nanocrystalline HAp can be recognized to its higher surface area, which in turn may lead to enhancements in fracture toughness and mechanical properties [92]. Moreover, it is anticipated that nHAp will exhibit superior bioactivity in comparison to HAp at the bulk, macro, and microscales [93]. In comparison to conventional HAp, nHAp demonstrates enhanced capabilities in terms of osteoblast adhesion, differentiation, and proliferation, resulting in accelerated bone regeneration within a condensed timeframe [94–96]. The nHAp exhibits exceptional surface characteristics, including a large surface area and roughness. These properties facilitate the attachment of cells and promote interaction with the host tissue, thereby enabling long-term functionality and efficient bone tissue engineering, which is a critical consideration [97, 98]. One of the primary factors associated with biomaterials is their notable surface area, which has a significant impact on cellular adhesion and enhanced cell density. Another crucial characteristic is the surface roughness, which acting a critical role in the interactions between implant and the host tissue. According to the findings of previous studies, cell-matrix interactions are thought to be aided by the surface qualities of biomaterials, and those important interactions are thought to take place within proximity of 1 nm from the consideration of the surface [97, 98].

8.6 EFFECTS OF NANOCRYSTALLAINE HYDROXYAPATITE ON BONE REGENERATION

According to research by Jahangirnezhad et al. [99], n-HAp has osteoconductive qualities that allow it to generate a substantial quantity of bone when used as a bone transplant. Similar findings were reported by Vullo et al. [100]. In the treatment of periodontal abnormalities in dogs, where n-HAp was shown to be both osteoconductive and osteoinductive. Jaw bone samples were used by Gotz et al. [101] to assess the immune histochemical characteristics of hydroxyapatite nanocrystalline silica gel. The research showed that n-HAp has biomimetic and osteoconductive capabilities. Human physiological bone turnover initially included these characteristics. Based on clinical outcomes that were on par with those seen with autogenously graft materials, the investigators came to the conclusion that n-HAp paste was appropriate for use in filling gaps in bones [102]. In addition, Zuev et al. [73] reported that the use of n-HAp paste for the treatment of periodontal osseous defects, which includes the treatment of periodontal abscesses, was not suitable. The combination of n-hydroxy acid and polylactic acid may be an excellent choice for the guided tissue regeneration (GTR) membrane as a graft material [103], as shown by research by Talal et al. [104] Though it functions as a barrier, this substance may improve bone repair by transporting biologically active molecules to the site of injury. Busen et al. [105] discovered that n-HAp was competitive with Bio-Oss in bone restoration procedures, lending credence to these findings. After four months, Bertobli et al. [106]. Investigated the quantity of bone development in Bio-Oss and n-HAp and found conflicting findings. Bone development was more in the Bio-Oss group than in the n-HAp group.

8.7 FUTURE PROSPECTIVE

The "Hydroxyapatite Market" study covers the years 2023–2031 and provides a thorough analysis of the market landscape, breaking down the global market into its component parts for companies operating in the North American, European, and Asian, South American, and African regions. The research provides organizations with an advantage in decision-making by providing a projection based on an analysis of the market's future prospects. In addition, the study analyses significant trends, facts, and information that is crucial to comprehending the market's development potential and provides insights into past and present market circumstances. It breaks down the industry by product and application and profiles the major companies in the field. Furthermore, the report presents comprehensive data regarding the compound annual growth rate (CAGR) status, revenue growth specifics, estimations of industry size and market share, as well as a detailed analysis of the segmentation of the hydroxyapatite market. This segmentation includes different types such as nano size powders and pastes (including TCP) and non-nano size pastes and powders (including TCP), and various applications including medical devices (bone regeneration), oral care (toothpaste, mouthwash), and other (food, pharma, research). Technological innovation and progress will contribute to the further enhancement of product performance, thereby facilitating its increased utilization in downstream applications. Understanding the hydroxyapatite market requires an examination of the market's dynamics (drivers, constraints, and opportunities), as well as the buying habits and preferences of consumers. The hydroxyapatite market has experienced a notable increase in value, rising from USD 633.6 million in 2017 to USD 2250.19 million in 2022. Based on the compound annual growth rate (CAGR), it is projected that this market will attain annual growth rate of 6.52% from 2023 to 2029 [106, 107].

8.8 CONCLUSION

This chapter gives a thorough look at how HAp is used in bone tissue and how nanocrystalline HAp affects bone regeneration. It discusses the synthesis methods of HAp, the uses of nanohydroxyapatite in the biomedical field, and the significance of appropriate ionic substitution to enhance the physical, mechanical, nadchemical properties of HAp. Various researchers extensively study certain ionic substitutions, but there is a scarcity of research on the incorporation of alternative ions that are not typically found in natural apatite. This presents intriguing challenges that warrant further investigation. To fully capitalize on the inherent advantages, it is imperative to possess a comprehensive comprehension of the desirable attributes associated with these ionic substitutions. Moreover, we are currently discussing the use of HAp particles with customized characteristics for potential applications in bone-tissue engineering and drug delivery. In conclusion, the report provides insights into the use of zinc, cobalt, and fluorine hydroxyapatite ions in bone tissue engineering. Additionally, it highlights potential avenues for further research in this field. In conclusion, HAp is a widely used material in various biomedical applications. However, we need to conduct additional research to enhance our understanding of HAp and its properties, especially regarding its suitability for long-term in vivo applications.

REFERENCES

1. L. L. Hench, "Bioceramics: from concept to clinic," *J. Am. Ceram. Soc.*, vol. 74, no. 7, pp. 1487–1510, Jul. 1991, doi: 10.1111/J.1151-2916.1991.TB07132.X.
2. M. Zandi et al., "Biocompatibility evaluation of nano-rod hydroxyapatite/gelatin coated with nano-HAp as a novel scaffold using mesenchymal stem cells," *Wiley Online Libr.*, vol. 92, no. 4, pp. 1244–1255, Mar. 2009, doi: 10.1002/jbm.a.32452.
3. S. Ghanaati et al., "The chemical composition of synthetic bone substitutes influences tissue reactions in vivo: histological and histomorphometrical analysis of the cellular inflammatory response to hydroxyapatite, beta-tricalcium phosphate and biphasic calcium phosphate ceramics," *Biomed. Mater.*, vol. 7, no. 1, p. 015005, Jan. 2012, doi: 10.1088/1748-6041/7/1/015005.
4. R. Murugan, S. R.-C. S. and Technology, and Undefined 2005, "Development of nanocomposites for bone grafting," *Elsevier*, Accessed: Jul. 17, 2023. [Online]. Available: https://www.sciencedirect.com/science/article/pii/S026635380500285X
5. S. Kapoor, U. Batra, S. Kohli, and R. Kumar, "Synthesis and characterization of zinc and fluorine co-substituted hydroxyapatite for bone and dental applications," *Mater. Today Proc.*, vol. 68, pp. 742–748, Jan. 2022, doi: 10.1016/J.MATPR.2022.06.051.
6. E. Boanini, M. Gazzano, A. B.-A. Biomaterialia, and Undefined 2010, "Ionic substitutions in calcium phosphates synthesized at low temperature," *Elsevier*, Accessed: Jul. 16, 2023. [Online]. Available: https://www.sciencedirect.com/science/article/pii/S1742706109005820
7. C. R. Gautam, S. Kumar, S. Biradar, S. Jose, and V. K. Mishra, "Synthesis and enhanced mechanical properties of MgO substituted hydroxyapatite: a bone substitute material," *RSC Adv.*, vol. 6, no. 72, pp. 67565–67574, Jul. 2016, doi: 10.1039/C6RA10839C.

8. C. Capuccini, P. Torricelli, E. Boanini, M. Gazzano, R. Giardino, and A. Bigi, "Interaction of Sr-doped hydroxyapatite nanocrystals with osteoclast and osteoblast-like cells," *J. Biomed. Mater. Res. Part A*, vol. 89A, no. 3, pp. 594–600, Jun. 2009, doi: 10.1002/JBM.A.31975.
9. B. Bracci, P. Torricelli, S. Panzavolta, E. Boanini, R. Giardino, and A. Bigi, "Effect of Mg^{2+}, Sr^{2+}, and Mn^{2+} on the chemico-physical and in vitro biological properties of calcium phosphate biomimetic coatings," *J. Inorg. Biochem.*, vol. 103, no. 12, pp. 1666–1674, Dec. 2009, doi: 10.1016/J.JINORGBIO.2009.09.009.
10. R. Z. LeGeros, "Biodegradation and bioresorption of calcium phosphate ceramics," *Clin. Mater.*, vol. 14, no. 1, pp. 65–88, Jan. 1993, doi: 10.1016/0267-6605(93)90049-D.
11. E. Landi, A. Tampieri, G. Celotti, S. Sprio, M. Sandri, and G. Logroscino, "Sr-substituted hydroxyapatites for osteoporotic bone replacement," *Acta Biomater.*, vol. 3, no. 6, pp. 961–969, Nov. 2007, doi: 10.1016/J.ACTBIO.2007.05.006.
12. "(2) (PDF) Development of zinc doped hydroxyapatite for bone implant applications" https://www.researchgate.net/publication/259621440_Development_of_Zinc_Doped_Hydroxyapatite_for_Bone_Implant_Applications (accessed Jul. 16, 2023).
13. A. Bianco, I. Cacciotti, M. Lombardi, and L. Montanaro, "Si-substituted hydroxyapatite nanopowders: synthesis, thermal stability and sinterability," *Mater. Res. Bull.*, vol. 44, no. 2, pp. 345–354, Feb. 2009, doi: 10.1016/J.MATERRESBULL.2008.05.013.
14. G. Singh, R. P. Singh, and S. S. Jolly, "Customized hydroxyapatites for bone-tissue engineering and drug delivery applications: a review," *J. Sol-Gel Sci. Technol.*, vol. 94, no. 3, pp. 505–530, Jan. 2020, doi: 10.1007/S10971-020-05222-1.
15. J. Ovesen, B. Møller-Madsen, J. S. Thomsen, G. Danscher, and L. Mosekilde, "The positive effects of zinc on skeletal strength in growing rats," *Bone*, vol. 29, no. 6, pp. 565–570, Dec. 2001, doi: 10.1016/S8756-3282(01)00616-0.
16. S. L. Hall, H. P. Dimai, and J. R. Farley, "Effects of zinc on human skeletal alkaline phosphatase activity in vitro," *Calcif. Tissue Int.*, vol. 64, no. 2, pp. 163–172, 1999.
17. "Role of zinc in bone formation and bone resorption - Yamaguchi - 1998 - The Journal of Trace Elements in Experimental Medicine - Wiley Online Library" https://onlinelibrary.wiley.com/doi/abs/10.1002/(SICI)1520-670X(1998)11:2/3%3C119::AID-JTRA5%3E3.0.CO;2-3 (accessed Jul. 16, 2023).
18. S. Miao et al., "Fabrication and evaluation of Zn containing fluoridated hydroxyapatite layer with Zn release ability," *Acta Biomater.*, vol. 4, no. 2, pp. 441–446, Mar. 2008, doi: 10.1016/J.ACTBIO.2007.08.013.
19. A. Bigi, E. Foresti, M. Gandolfi, M. Gazzano, and N. Roveri, "Isomorphous substitutions in β-tricalcium phosphate: the different effects of zinc and strontium," *J. Inorg. Biochem.*, vol. 66, no. 4, pp. 259–265, Jun. 1997, doi: 10.1016/S0162-0134(96)00219-X.
20. O. Kaygili and C. Tatar, "The investigation of some physical properties and microstructure of Zn-doped hydroxyapatite bioceramics prepared by sol-gel method," *J. Sol-Gel Sci. Technol.*, vol. 61, no. 2, pp. 296–309, Feb. 2012.
21. E. Jallot, J. Nedelec, A. Grimault, … E. C.-C. and surfaces B., and Undefined 2005, "STEM and EDXS characterisation of physico-chemical reactions at the periphery of sol–gel derived Zn-substituted hydroxyapatites during interactions with biological," *Elsevier*, Accessed: Jul. 16, 2023. [Online]. Available: https://www.sciencedirect.com/science/article/pii/S092777650500086X

22. M. Yamaguchi, H. Oishi, and Y. Suketa, "Stimulatory effect of zinc on bone formation in tissue culture," *Biochem. Pharmacol.*, vol. 36, no. 22, pp. 4007–4012, Nov. 1987, doi: 10.1016/0006-2952(87)90471-0.
23. A. Ito, K. Ojima, H. Naito, N. Ichinose, and T. Tateishi, "Preparation, solubility, and cytocompatibility of zinc-releasing calcium phosphate ceramics," *J. Biomed. Mater. Res.*, vol. 50, no. 2, pp. 178–183, 2000, doi: 10.1002/(SICI)1097-4636(200005)50:2<178::AID-JBM12>3.0.CO;2-5.
24. M. Yamaguchi, "Role of zinc in bone formation and bone resorption," *J. Trace Elem. Exp. Med.*, vol. 11, no. 23, pp. 119–135, 1998, doi: 10.1002/(sici)1520-670x(1998)11:2/3<119::aid-jtra5>3.3.co;2-s.
25. G. Ps, "Biological evaluation of biomaterials for bone tissue regeneration," 2011.
26. J. H. Shepherd, D. V. Shepherd, and S. M. Best, "Substituted hydroxyapatites for bone repair," *J. Mater. Sci. Mater. Med.*, vol. 23, no. 10, pp. 2335–2347, Oct. 2012, doi: 10.1007/S10856-012-4598-2.
27. A. Camaioni, I. Cacciotti, L. Campagnolo, and A. Bianco, "Silicon-substituted hydroxyapatite for biomedical applications," *Hydroxyapatite Biomed. Appl.*, pp. 343–373, Jan. 2015, doi: 10.1016/B978-1-78242-033-0.00015-8.
28. A. M. Pietak, J. W. Reid, M. J. Stott, and M. Sayer, "Silicon substitution in the calcium phosphate bioceramics," *Biomaterials*, vol. 28, no. 28, pp. 4023–4032, Oct. 2007, doi: 10.1016/J.BIOMATERIALS.2007.05.003.
29. I. Cacciotti, "Cationic and anionic substitutions in hydroxyapatite," *Handb. Bioceram. Biocomposites*, pp. 145–211, Jan. 2016.
30. Y. Qiao et al., "Stimulation of bone growth following zinc incorporation into biomaterials," *Biomaterials*, vol. 35, no. 25, pp. 6882–6897, Aug. 2014, doi: 10.1016/J.BIOMATERIALS.2014.04.101.
31. I. Uysal, F. Severcan, A. Tezcaner, and Z. Evis, "Co-doping of hydroxyapatite with zinc and fluoride improves mechanical and biological properties of hydroxyapatite," *Prog. Nat. Sci. Mater. Int.*, vol. 24, no. 4, pp. 340–349, 2014, doi: 10.1016/J.PNSC.2014.06.004.
32. H. Qu and M. Wei, "The effect of fluoride contents in fluoridated hydroxyapatite on osteoblast behavior," *Acta Biomater.*, vol. 2, no. 1, pp. 113–119, Jan. 2006, doi: 10.1016/J.ACTBIO.2005.09.003.
33. J. M. Ten Cate and J. D. B. Featherstone, "Mechanistic aspects of the interactions between fluoride and dental enamel," *Crit. Rev. Oral Biol. Med.*, vol. 2, no. 3, pp. 283–296, Jul. 1991, doi: 10.1177/10454411910020030101.
34. R. Z. Legeros, L. M. Silverstone, G. Daculsi, and L. M. Kerebel, "In vitro caries-like lesion formation in F-containing tooth enamel," *J. Dent. Res.*, vol. 62, no. 2, pp. 138–144, Feb. 1983, doi: 10.1177/00220345830620021101.
35. H. Qu and M. Wei, "Synthesis and characterization of fluorine-containing hydroxyapatite by a pH-cycling method," *J. Mater. Sci. Mater. Med.*, vol. 16, no. 2, pp. 129–133, Feb. 2005.
36. Y. Chen and X. Miao, "Thermal and chemical stability of fluorohydroxyapatite ceramics with different fluorine contents," *Biomaterials*, vol. 26, no. 11, pp. 1205–1210, Apr. 2005, doi: 10.1016/J.BIOMATERIALS.2004.04.027.
37. C. Y. C. Pak, J. E. Zerwekh, and P. Antich, "Anabolic effects of fluoride on bone," *Trends Endocrinol. Metab.*, vol. 6, no. 7, pp. 229–234, 1995, doi: 10.1016/1043-2760(95)00111-T.

38. J. R. Farley, N. Tarbaux, S. Hall, and D. J. Baylink, "Evidence that fluoride-stimulated 3[H]-thymidine incorporation in embryonic chick calvarial cell cultures is dependent on the presence of a bone cell mitogen, sensitive to changes in the phosphate concentration, and modulated by systemic skeletal effectors," *Metabolism*, vol. 37, no. 10, pp. 988–995, 1988, doi: 10.1016/0026-0495(88)90158-8.
39. U. K. Bhawal, H. J. Lee, K. Arikawa, M. Shimosaka, M. Suzuki, T. Toyama, T. Sato, R. Kawamata, C. Taguchi, N. Hamada, I. Nasu, H. Arakawa and K. Shibutani, "Micromolar sodium fluoride mediates anti-osteoclastogenesis in porphyromonas gingivalis-induced alveolar bone loss," *Int. J. Oral Sci.*, vol. 7, no. 4, pp. 242–249, 2015, doi: 10.1038/IJOS.2015.28.
40. M. Prakasam, J. Locs, K. Salma-Ancane, D. Loca, A. Largeteau, and L. Berzina-Cimdina, "Functional biomaterials fabrication, properties and applications of dense hydroxyapatite: a review," *J. Funct. Biomater*, vol. 6, pp. 1099–1140, 2015, doi: 10.3390/jfb6041099.
41. W. Fan, R. Crawford, and Y. Xiao, "Enhancing in vivo vascularized bone formation by cobalt chloride-treated bone marrow stromal cells in a tissue engineered periosteum model," *Biomaterials*, vol. 31, no. 13, pp. 3580–3589, May 2010, doi: 10.1016/J.BIOMATERIALS.2010.01.083.
42. C. Wu, Y. Zhou, W. Fan, P. Han, J. Chang, J. Yuen, M. Zhang and Y. Xiao, "Hypoxia-mimicking mesoporous bioactive glass scaffolds with controllable cobalt ion release for bone tissue engineering," *Biomaterials*, vol. 33, no. 7, pp. 2076–2085, Mar. 2012, doi: 10.1016/J.BIOMATERIALS.2011.11.042.
43. Z. Lu, B. Wang, Y. Hu, W. Liu, Y. Zhao, R. Yang, Z. Li, J. Luo, B. Chi, Z. Jiang, M. Li, S. Mu, S. Liao, J. Zhang and X. Sun, "An isolated zinc–cobalt atomic pair for highly active and durable oxygen reduction," *Angew. Chemie Int. Ed.*, vol. 58, no. 9, pp. 2622–2626, Feb. 2019, doi: 10.1002/ANIE.201810175.
44. M. M. Azevedo, G. Jell, M. D. O'Donnell, R. V. Law, R. G. Hill, and M. M. Stevens, "Synthesis and characterization of hypoxia-mimicking bioactive glasses for skeletal regeneration," *J. Mater. Chem.*, vol. 20, no. 40, pp. 8854–8864, Oct. 2010, doi: 10.1039/C0JM01111H.
45. A. Kahaie Khosrowshahi, A. B. Khoshfetrat, Y. B. Khosrowshahi, and H. Maleki-Ghaleh, "Cobalt content modulates characteristics and osteogenic properties of cobalt-containing hydroxyapatite in in-vitro milieu," *Mater. Today Commun.*, vol. 27, no. April, p. 102392, 2021, doi: 10.1016/j.mtcomm.2021.102392.
46. C. Moseke and U. Gbureck, "Tetracalcium phosphate: synthesis, properties and biomedical applications," *Acta Biomater.*, vol. 6, no. 10, pp. 3815–3823, Oct. 2010, doi: 10.1016/J.ACTBIO.2010.04.020.
47. S. I. Stupp and G. W. Ciegler, "Organoapatites: materials for artificial bone. I. synthesis and microstructure," *J. Biomed. Mater. Res.*, vol. 26, no. 2, pp. 169–183, Feb. 1992, doi: 10.1002/JBM.820260204.
48. S. V. Dorozhkin, "Nanodimensional and nanocrystalline apatites and other calcium orthophosphates in biomedical engineering, biology and medicine," *Materials (Basel).*, vol. 2, no. 4, pp. 1975–2045, 2009, doi: 10.3390/MA2041975.
49. S. V. Dorozhkin, "Nanosized and nanocrystalline calcium orthophosphates," *Acta Biomater.*, vol. 6, no. 3, pp. 715–734, Mar. 2010, doi: 10.1016/J.ACTBIO.2009.10.031.
50. A. J. Wagoner Johnson and B. A. Herschler, "A review of the mechanical behavior of CaP and CaP/polymer composites for applications in bone replacement and repair," *Acta Biomater.*, vol. 7, no. 1, pp. 16–30, 2011, doi: 10.1016/J.ACTBIO.2010.07.012.

51. S. Liu, H. Zhou, H. Liu, H. Ji, W. Fei, and E. Luo, "Fluorine-contained hydroxyapatite suppresses bone resorption through inhibiting osteoclasts differentiation and function in vitro and in vivo," *Cell Prolif.*, vol. 52, no. 3, 2019, doi: 10.1111/cpr.12613.
52. M. Sadat-Shojai, M. T. Khorasani, E. Dinpanah-Khoshdargi, and A. Jamshidi, "Synthesis methods for nanosized hydroxyapatite with diverse structures," *Acta Biomater.*, vol. 9, no. 8, pp. 7591–7621, 2013, doi: 10.1016/J.ACTBIO.2013.04.012.
53. B. L. Cushing, V. L. Kolesnichenko, and C. J. O'Connor, "Recent advances in the liquid-phase syntheses of inorganic nanoparticles," *Chem. Rev.*, vol. 104, no. 9, pp. 3893–3946, Sep. 2004, doi: 10.1021/CR030027B.
54. O. Kaygili and C. Tatar, "The investigation of some physical properties and microstructure of Zn-doped hydroxyapatite bioceramics prepared by sol-gel method", *J. Sol-Gel Sci. Technol.*, vol. 61, pp. 296–309, 2012, doi: 10.1007/s10971-011-2627-0.
55. H. Eshtiagh-Hosseini, M. R. Housaindokht, and M. Chahkandi, "Effects of parameters of sol–gel process on the phase evolution of sol–gel-derived hydroxyapatite," *Mater. Chem. Phys.*, vol. 106, no. 2–3, pp. 310–316, Dec. 2007, doi: 10.1016/J.MATCHEMPHYS.2007.06.002.
56. A. Naqshbandi, I. Sopyan, Gunawan, and Suryanto, "Sol-gel synthesis of Zn doped HA powders and their conversion to porous bodies," *Appl. Mech. Mater.*, vol. 493, pp. 603–608, 2014, doi: 10.4028/WWW.SCIENTIFIC.NET/AMM.493.603.
57. C. C. Negrila, M. V. Predoi, S. L. Iconaru, and D. Predoi, "Development of zinc-doped hydroxyapatite by sol-gel method for medical applications," *Molecules*, vol. 23, no. 11, Nov. 2018, doi: 10.3390/MOLECULES23112986.
58. E. Fujii, M. Ohkubo, K. Tsuru, S. Hayakawa, A. Osaka, K. Kawabata, C. Bonhomme and F. Babonneau, "Selective protein adsorption property and characterization of nanocrystalline zinc-containing hydroxyapatite," *Acta Biomater.*, vol. 2, no. 1, pp. 69–74, Jan. 2006, doi: 10.1016/J.ACTBIO.2005.09.002.
59. E. S. Thian, T. Konishi, Y. Kawanobe, P. N. Lim, C. Choong, B. Ho, and M. Aizawa, "Zinc-substituted hydroxyapatite: a biomaterial with enhanced bioactivity and antibacterial properties," *J. Mater. Sci. Mater. Med.*, vol. 24, no. 2, pp. 437–445, Feb. 2013, doi: 10.1007/S10856-012-4817-X.
60. F. Ren, R. Xin, X. Ge, and Y. Leng, "Characterization and structural analysis of zinc-substituted hydroxyapatites," *Acta Biomater.*, vol. 5, no. 8, pp. 3141–3149, Oct. 2009, doi: 10.1016/J.ACTBIO.2009.04.014.
61. S. C. Cox, P. Jamshidi, L. M. Grover, and K. K. Mallick, "Preparation and characterisation of nanophase Sr, Mg, and Zn substituted hydroxyapatite by aqueous precipitation," *Mater. Sci. Eng. C. Mater. Biol. Appl.*, vol. 35, no. 1, pp. 106–114, 2014, doi: 10.1016/J.MSEC.2013.10.015.
62. M. Ashuri, F. Moztarzadeh, N. Nezafati, A. Ansari Hamedani, and M. Tahriri, "Development of a composite based on hydroxyapatite and magnesium and zinc-containing sol–gel-derived bioactive glass for bone substitute applications," *Mater. Sci. Eng. C*, vol. 32, no. 8, pp. 2330–2339, Dec. 2012, doi: 10.1016/J.MSEC.2012.07.004.
63. B. G. Rao, D. Mukherjee, and B. M. Reddy, "Novel approaches for preparation of nanoparticles," *Nanostructures Nov. Ther. Synth. Charact. Appl.*, pp. 1–36, Jan. 2017, doi: 10.1016/B978-0-323-46142-9.00001-3.
64. Z. Stojanović, L. Veselinović, S. Marković, N. Ignjatović, and D. Uskoković, "Hydrothermal synthesis of nanosized pure and cobalt-exchanged hydroxyapatite," *Mater. Manuf. Process.*, vol. 24, no. 10–11, pp. 1096–1103, Oct. 2009, doi: 10.1080/10426910903032113.

65. Ž. Radovanović et al., "Biocompatibility and antimicrobial activity of zinc(II)-doped hydroxyapatite, synthesized by a hydrothermal method," *J. Serbian Chem. Soc.*, vol. 77, no. 12, pp. 1787–1798, 2012, doi: 10.2298/JSC121019131R.
66. M. Li, X. Xiao, R. Liu, C. Chen, and L. Huang, "Structural characterization of zinc-substituted hydroxyapatite prepared by hydrothermal method," *J. Mater. Sci. Mater. Med.*, vol. 19, no. 2, pp. 797–803, Feb. 2008, doi: 10.1007/S10856-007-3213-4.
67. Y. Hattori, H. Mori, J. Chou, and M. Otsuka, "Mechanochemical synthesis of zinc-apatitic calcium phosphate and the controlled zinc release for bone tissue engineering," vol. 42, no. 4, pp. 595–601, Jan. 2016, doi: 10.3109/03639045.2015.1061537.
68. L. Boyer, J. Carpena, and J. L. Lacout, "Synthesis of phosphate-silicate apatites at atmospheric pressure," *Solid State Ionics*, vol. 95, no. 1–2, pp. 121–129, Feb. 1997, doi: 10.1016/S0167-2738(96)00571-1.
69. K. S. Leshkivich and E. A. Monroe, "Solubility characteristics of synthetic silicate sulphate apatites," *J. Mater. Sci.*, vol. 28, no. 1, pp. 9–14, Jan. 1993.
70. B. D. Hahn et al., "Aerosol deposition of silicon-substituted hydroxyapatite coatings for biomedical applications," *Thin Solid Films*, vol. 518, no. 8, pp. 2194–2199, Feb. 2010, doi: 10.1016/J.TSF.2009.09.024.
71. S. Mann, "Biomineralization: principles and concepts in bioinorganic materials chemistry," 2001, Accessed: Jul. 03, 2023. [Online]. Available: https://books.google.com/books?hl=en&lr=&id=YLNl5Jm7XxwC&oi=fnd&pg=PA1&ots=LqeT-nyPOH&sig=zb_BnFc9QMUcCWTFKDoL4zTfzUw.
72. S. Kanaya, E. Nemoto, Y. Sakisaka, and H. Shimauchi, "Calcium-mediated increased expression of fibroblast growth factor-2 acts through NF-κB and PGE2/EP4 receptor signaling pathways in cementoblasts," *Bone*, vol. 56, no. 2, pp. 398–405, Oct. 2013, doi: 10.1016/J.BONE.2013.06.031.
73. C. Yang, J. S. Lee, U. W. Jung, Y. K. Seo, J. K. Park, and S. H. Choi, "Periodontal regeneration with nano-hyroxyapatite-coated silk scaffolds in dogs," *J. Periodontal Implant Sci.*, vol. 43, no. 6, pp. 315–322, Dec. 2013, doi: 10.5051/JPIS.2013.43.6.315.
74. R. G. Saleh, O. M. Gab Allah, H. M. E. Tokhey, and H. M. El-Guindy, "Evaluation of hydroxyapatite nanoparticles with and without silver nanoparticles in the treatment of induced periodontitis in dogs," *J. Am. Sci.*, vol. 10, no. 12, pp. 21–33, Dec. 2014.
75. H. Shahoon, R. Hamedi, Z. Yadegari, and V. M. Hosseiny, "The comparison of silver and hydroxyapatite nanoparticles biocompatibility on L929 fibroblast cells: an," 2013, doi: 10.4172/2157-7439.1000173.
76. W. Sun, C. Chu, J. Wang, and H. Zhao, "Comparison of periodontal ligament cells responses to dense and nanophase hydroxyapatite," *J. Mater. Sci. Mater. Med.*, vol. 18, no. 5, pp. 677–683, May 2007, doi: 10.1007/S10856-006-0019-8.
77. E. S. Thian, J. Huang, Z. Ahmad, M. J. Edirisinghe, S. N. Jayasinghe, D. C. Ireland, R. A. Brooks, N. Rushton, S. M. Best, and W. Bonfield, "Influence of nanohydroxyapatite patterns deposited by electrohydrodynamic spraying on osteoblast response," *J. Biomed. Mater. Res. - Part A*, vol. 85, no. 1, pp. 188–194, Apr. 2008, doi: 10.1002/JBM.A.31564.
78. A. Pilloni, G. Pompa, M. Saccucci, G. D. Carlo, L. Rimondini, M. Brama, B. Zeza, F. Wannenes, and S. Migliaccio, "Analysis of human alveolar osteoblast behavior on a nano-hydroxyapatite substrate: an in vitro study," *BMC Oral Health*, vol. 14, no. 1, Mar. 2014, doi: 10.1186/1472-6831-14-22.

79. T. J. Webster, C. Ergun, R. H. Doremus, R. W. Siegel, and R. Bizios, "Enhanced functions of osteoblasts on nanophase ceramics," *Biomaterials*, vol. 21, no. 17, pp. 1803–1810, Sep. 2000, doi: 10.1016/S0142-9612(00)00075-2.
80. X. Liu, M. Zhao, J. Lu, J. Ma, J. Wei, and S. Wei, "Cell responses to two kinds of nanohydroxyapatite with different sizes and crystallinities," *Int. J. Nanomedicine*, vol. 7, pp. 1239–1250, 2012, doi: 10.2147/IJN.S28098.
81. M. F. Hsieh, J. K. L. Li, C. A. J. Lin, S. H. Huang, R. A. Sperling, W. J. Parak, and W. H. Chang, "Tracking of cellular uptake of hydrophilic CdSe/ZnS quantum dots/hydroxyapatite composites nanoparticles in MC3T3-E1 osteoblast cells," *J. Nanosci. Nanotechnol.*, vol. 9, no. 4, pp. 2758–2762, Apr. 2009, doi: 10.1166/JNN.2009.463.
82. R. Detsch, D. Hagmeyer, M. Neumann, S. Schaefer, A. Vortkamp, M. Wuelling, G. Ziegler, and M. Epple, "The resorption of nanocrystalline calcium phosphates by osteoclast-like cells," *Acta Biomater.*, vol. 6, no. 8, pp. 3223–3233, 2010, doi: 10.1016/J.ACTBIO.2010.03.003.
83. M. Motskin, D.M. Wright, K. Muller, N. Kyle, T.G. Gard, A.E. Porter, and J.N. Skepper, "Hydroxyapatite nano and microparticles: correlation of particle properties with cytotoxicity and biostability," *Biomaterials*, vol. 30, no. 19, pp. 3307–3317, Jul. 2009, doi: 10.1016/J.BIOMATERIALS.2009.02.044.
84. B. Lowe, J. G. Hardy, and L. J. Walsh, "Optimizing nanohydroxyapatite nanocomposites for bone tissue engineering," *ACS Omega*, vol. 5, no. 1, pp. 1–9, Jan. 2020.
85. K. J. L. Burg, S. Porter, and J. F. Kellam, "Biomaterial developments for bone tissue engineering," *Biomaterials*, vol. 21, no. 23, pp. 2347–2359, Dec. 2000, doi: 10.1016/S0142-9612(00)00102-2.
86. H. Zhou and J. Lee, "Nanoscale hydroxyapatite particles for bone tissue engineering," *Acta Biomater.*, vol. 7, no. 7, pp. 2769–2781, Jul. 2011, doi: 10.1016/J.ACTBIO.2011.03.019.
87. N. Kantharia, S. Naik, S. Apte, M. Kheur, S. Kheur, and B. Kale, "Nano-hydroxyapatite and its contemporary applications," *J. Dent. Res. Sci. Dev.*, vol. 1, no. 1, p. 15, 2014, doi: 10.4103/2348-3407.126135.
88. B. Palazzo, M. Iafisco, M. Laforgia, N. Margiotta, G. Natile, C. L. Bianchi, D. Walsh, S. Mann, and N. Roveri, "Biomimetic hydroxyapatite–drug nanocrystals as potential bone substitutes with antitumor drug delivery properties," *Adv. Funct. Mater.*, vol. 17, no. 13, pp. 2180–2188, Sep. 2007, doi: 10.1002/ADFM.200600361.
89. K. Deshmukh, M. M. Shaik, S. R. Ramanan, and M. Kowshik, "Self-activated fluorescent hydroxyapatite nanoparticles: a promising agent for bioimaging and biolabeling," *ACS Biomater. Sci. Eng.*, vol. 2, no. 8, pp. 1257–1264, Aug. 2016.
90. C. Verwilghen, S. Rio, A. Nzihou, D. Gauthier, G. Flamant, and P. J. Sharrock, "Preparation of high specific surface area hydroxyapatite for environmental applications," *J. Mater. Sci.*, vol. 42, no. 15, pp. 6062–6066, Aug. 2007.
91. M. T. Elsayed, A. A. Hassan, S. A. Abdelaal, M. M. Taher, M. khalaf Ahmed, and K. R. Shoueir, "Morphological, antibacterial, and cell attachment of cellulose acetate nanofibers containing modified hydroxyapatite for wound healing utilizations," *J. Mater. Res. Technol.*, vol. 9, no. 6, pp. 13927–13936, Nov. 2020, doi: 10.1016/J.JMRT.2020.09.094.
92. R. Z. LeGeros, "Biodegradation and bioresorption of calcium phosphate ceramics," *Clin. Mater.*, vol. 14, no. 1, pp. 65–88, 1993, doi: 10.1016/0267-6605(93)90049-D.

93. T. J. Webster, C. Ergun, R. H. Doremus, R. W. Siegel, and R. Bizios, "Enhanced functions of osteoblasts on nanophase ceramics," *Biomaterials*, vol. 21, no. 17, pp. 1803–1810, Sep. 2000, doi: 10.1016/S0142-9612(00)00075-2.
94. H. M. Kim, T. Himeno, M. Kawashita, T. Kokubo, and T. Nakamura, "The mechanism of biomineralization of bone-like apatite on synthetic hydroxyapatite: an in vitro assessment," *J. R. Soc. Interface*, vol. 1, no. 1, pp. 17–22, Nov. 2004, doi: 10.1098/RSIF.2004.0003.
95. P. N. Chavan, M. M. Bahir, R. U. Mene, M. P. Mahabole, and R. S. Khairnar, "Study of nanobiomaterial hydroxyapatite in simulated body fluid: formation and growth of apatite," *Mater. Sci. Eng. B*, vol. 168, no. 1–3, pp. 224–230, Apr. 2010, doi: 10.1016/J.MSEB.2009.11.012.
96. T. S. Srivatsan, "*Biomaterials: a nano approach*, by Sreeram Ramakrishna, Murugan Ramalingam, T. S. Sampath Kumar, and Winston O. Soboyejo," *J. Manuf. Process.*, vol. 29, no. 11–12, pp. 1510–1511, Dec. 2014, doi: 10.1080/10426914.2014.950068.
97. M. Sadat-Shojai, M. T. Khorasani, E. Dinpanah-Khoshdargi, and A. Jamshidi, "Synthesis methods for nanosized hydroxyapatite with diverse structures," *Acta Biomater.*, vol. 9, no. 8, pp. 7591–7621, Aug. 2013, doi: 10.1016/J.ACTBIO.2013.04.012.
98. M. Jahangirnezhad, S. Amirpoor, M. Rahimzadeh Larki, and A. Jundi Shapour, "The effects of Nanohydroxyapatite on bone regeneration in rat calvarial defects," *usa-journals.com*, vol. 1, no. 4, 2013, Accessed: Jul. 10, 2023. [Online]. Available: http://www.usa-journals.com/wp-content/uploads/2013/03/Jahangirnezhad_Vol14.pdf
99. C. Vullo, M. C. T. Meligrana, G. Rossi, A. M. Tambella, F. Dini, P. A. Palumbo, and A. Spaterna, "Use of nanohydroxyapatite in regenerative therapy in dogs affected by periodontopathy: preliminary results," *Annals Clin. Lab Res.* vol. 3, no. 2:18, pp. 1–6, Jan. 2015.
100. W. Götz, T. Gerber, B. Michel, S. Lossdörfer, K. O. Henkel, and F. Heinemann, "Immunohistochemical characterization of nanocrystalline hydroxyapatite silica gel (NanoBone(r)) osteogenesis: a study on biopsies from human jaws," *Clin. Oral Implants Res.*, vol. 19, no. 10, pp. 1016–1026, Oct. 2008, doi: 10.1111/J.1600-0501.2008.01569.X.
101. F. X. Huber, N. McArthur, J. Hillmeier, H. J. Kock, M. Baier, M. Diwo, I. Berger, and P. J. Meeder, "Void filling of tibia compression fracture zones using a novel resorbable nanocrystalline hydroxyapatite paste in combination with a hydroxyapatite ceramic core: first clinical results," *Arch. Orthop. Trauma Surg.*, vol. 126, no. 8, pp. 533–540, Oct. 2006, doi: 10.1007/S00402-006-0170-1.
102. G. Zimmermann and A. Moghaddam, "Allograft bone matrix versus synthetic bone graft substitutes," *Injury*, vol. 42, no. SUPPL. 2, Sep. 2011, doi: 10.1016/j.injury.2011.06.199.
103. A. Talal, I. J. McKay, K. E. Tanner, and F. J. Hughes, "Effects of hydroxyapatite and PDGF concentrations on osteoblast growth in a nanohydroxyapatite-polylactic acid composite for guided tissue regeneration," *J. Mater. Sci. Mater. Med.*, vol. 24, no. 9, pp. 2211–2221, Sep. 2013, doi: 10.1007/S10856-013-4963-9.
104. D. Busenlechner, C. D. Huber, C. Vasak, A. Dobsak, R. Gruber, and G. Watzek, "Sinus augmentation analysis revised: the gradient of graft consolidation," *Clin. Oral Implants Res.*, vol. 20, no. 10, pp. 1078–1083, Oct. 2009, doi: 10.1111/J.1600-0501.2009.01733.X.
105. V. Lekovic, P. M. Camargo, M. Weinlaender, N. Vasilic, and E. B. Kenney, "Comparison of platelet-rich plasma, bovine porous bone mineral, and guided tissue regeneration

versus platelet-rich plasma and bovine porous bone mineral in the treatment of intrabony defects: a reentry study," *J. Periodontol.*, vol. 73, no. 2, pp. 198–205, Feb. 2002, doi: 10.1902/jop.2002.73.2.198.

106. "2023 Hydroxyapatite Market Recent Industry Scope, Future Trends and Growth Forecast by 2030 - MarketWatch."

107. "2023 Hydroxyapatite Market Outlook Report - Market Size, Market Split, Market Shares Data, Insights, Trends, Opportunities, Companies: Growth Forecasts by Product Type, Application, and Region from 2022 to 2030." https://www.researchandmarkets.com/reports/5688605/2023-hydroxyapatite-market-outlook-report (accessed Jul. 10, 2023).

9 Calcium Phosphate-Based Biomaterials for Drug Delivery in Bone Tissue Engineering

Dhruv Bhatnagar and Sanjeev Gautam
Advanced Functional Materials Laboratory, Dr. S.S. Bhatnagar University Institute of Chemical Engineering and Technology, Panjab University, Chandigarh, India

9.1 INTRODUCTION

Calcium phosphate-based biomaterials have emerged as a promising avenue for drug delivery in bone tissue engineering, revolutionizing the treatment of bone defects and fractures. The field of bone tissue engineering aims to repair and regenerate damaged bone tissue using biomaterials that can interact with the body's natural processes and support cellular growth [1]. Among the diverse range of biomaterials available, calcium phosphate-based materials have garnered significant attention due to their exceptional biocompatibility, osteoconductivity, and ability to degrade gradually over time, allowing for controlled drug release [2]. In this article, we will explore the key features of calcium phosphate-based biomaterials, their advantages for drug delivery, and the potential applications and challenges in the field of bone tissue engineering. The biocompatibility of calcium phosphate-based biomaterials is fundamental to their successful application in bone tissue engineering [3,4]. Biocompatibility refers to the ability of a material to interact with living tissues without causing harmful effects or eliciting an adverse immune response. Calcium phosphate materials, particularly hydroxyapatite and tricalcium phosphate, possess a chemical composition similar to the mineral component of natural bone [5]. This similarity allows these biomaterials to integrate seamlessly with the surrounding bone tissue, providing an excellent platform for bone regeneration. When implanted into the body, the biomaterials do not trigger rejection or inflammation, making them ideal candidates for drug delivery systems in bone tissue engineering [6]. Osteoconductivity is another critical aspect of calcium phosphate-based biomaterials that makes them suitable for

DOI: 10.1201/9781003360605-9

bone tissue engineering. Osteoconductivity refers to the ability of a biomaterial to support the attachment, proliferation, and differentiation of bone-forming cells, such as osteoblasts [7]. Calcium phosphate materials provide a favorable surface for cell adhesion, promoting cell migration and colonization at the implant site. As a result, these materials facilitate the formation of new bone tissue, aiding in the repair of bone defects or fractures. The osteoconductivity of calcium phosphate-based biomaterials is instrumental in promoting successful tissue regeneration and functional restoration [8].

The advantage of using calcium phosphate-based biomaterials for drug delivery in bone tissue engineering is their capability to serve as drug carriers, facilitating localized and controlled drug release [9]. Incorporating bioactive molecules or therapeutic agents into the biomaterials enables the delivery of drugs directly to the implant site, avoiding the need for systemic administration. This localized drug delivery approach minimizes the risk of systemic side effects and enhances the therapeutic efficacy of the treatment [10]. Furthermore, by controlling the drug release rate and duration, these biomaterials can create a conducive environment for bone regeneration, supporting cell proliferation and differentiation. Various drugs can be incorporated, such as growth factors to stimulate bone growth, anti-inflammatory agents to reduce swelling, and antimicrobial agents to prevent infection [11]. This multifunctional approach contributes to better outcomes in bone tissue engineering. The scaffold function of calcium phosphate-based biomaterials also plays a crucial role in facilitating drug delivery and promoting bone regeneration [12]. The biomaterial scaffold provides mechanical support and a 3D structure that guides cell growth and tissue formation. By loading drugs onto the scaffold, the biomaterial can act as a carrier and reservoir for the therapeutic agents, ensuring their controlled and sustained release over time [13]. The scaffold allows the drugs to be in close proximity to the target cells, maximizing their impact on the regenerative process. Additionally, the scaffold's porous nature allows for cell infiltration and nutrient diffusion, creating an environment conducive to cellular activity and tissue regeneration [14]. The gradual degradation of calcium phosphate-based biomaterials is a key factor in their drug delivery capabilities. These biomaterials can degrade over time, coinciding with the healing process of the bone tissue [15]. As the biomaterial degrades, it releases the incorporated drugs, providing a continuous and localized supply of therapeutic agents at the implant site. This controlled drug release ensures that the drugs are available when and where they are needed most during the tissue regeneration process [16]. The rate of degradation can be adjusted to match the rate of bone formation, ensuring optimal drug delivery throughout the healing period. This feature sets calcium phosphate-based biomaterials apart as an ideal choice for drug delivery in bone tissue engineering [17].

Moreover, the versatility of calcium phosphate-based biomaterials allows for various forms to be used in drug delivery strategies. These biomaterials can be fabricated as porous scaffolds, microspheres, or nanoparticles, each offering distinct advantages in drug delivery [18]. Porous scaffolds provide a large surface area for drug loading and allow for the incorporation of different drugs at different locations within the scaffold. Microspheres and nanoparticles offer increased surface-to-volume ratios, enabling more precise control over drug release kinetics [19, 20]. This diversity of forms ensures that the most suitable drug delivery system can be selected for specific bone tissue engineering applications [21]. Calcium phosphate-based biomaterials can be combined with bone-forming cells, such as mesenchymal stem cells (MSCs), to further enhance bone tissue regeneration. The drug-loaded biomaterial scaffold provides a supportive environment for the viability, proliferation, and differentiation of MSCs [22]. These cells can then differentiate into osteoblasts, contributing directly to the formation of new bone tissue [23]. The synergy between drug delivery and cell-based therapy improves the overall regenerative potential of calcium phosphate-based biomaterials, making them an exciting avenue for advancing bone tissue engineering techniques [24]. While calcium phosphate-based biomaterials hold tremendous potential for drug delivery in bone tissue engineering, there are challenges that need to be addressed. One such challenge is achieving precise control over drug release kinetics [25]. The rate of degradation and drug release should be carefully optimized to ensure that the drugs are delivered at the right concentration and time to facilitate bone regeneration without causing adverse effects. Additionally, the design and fabrication of biomaterial scaffolds need to consider the mechanical properties necessary to withstand physiological loads during the healing process [26]. Ensuring the mechanical stability of the scaffold is crucial for the success of the implant and the subsequent tissue regeneration [15].

Calcium phosphate-based biomaterials have emerged as a game-changer in the field of bone tissue engineering, particularly for drug delivery applications. Their biocompatibility, osteoconductivity, and ability to degrade gradually make them an ideal choice for promoting bone regeneration [27]. By incorporating drugs into these biomaterials, localized and controlled drug delivery can be achieved, enhancing the therapeutic outcomes while minimizing systemic side effects. Its versatile forms and potential combination with bone-forming cells, calcium phosphate-based biomaterials offer a promising approach to revolutionize the treatment of bone defects and fractures, contributing to improved patient outcomes and quality of life [28]. Despite the challenges, continued research and development in this area hold the potential to transform the landscape of bone tissue engineering and drug delivery in the future.

9.2 FABRICATION METHODS OF CALCIUM PHOSPHATE-BASED DRUG DELIVERY SYSTEMS

Fabrication methods for calcium phosphate-based drug delivery systems are essential for tailoring the properties of the biomaterials and optimizing drug release characteristics. Various techniques have been developed to incorporate drugs into calcium phosphate matrices and create drug-loaded systems suitable for bone tissue engineering applications as shown in Figure 9.1. Fabrication methods for calcium phosphate-based drug delivery systems primarily involve electrospinning and the sol-gel method. These fabrication methods offer different advantages and are chosen based on the specific requirements of the drug delivery system [29]. By carefully selecting the appropriate fabrication technique, researchers can optimize the drug release kinetics, mechanical properties, and structural features of calcium

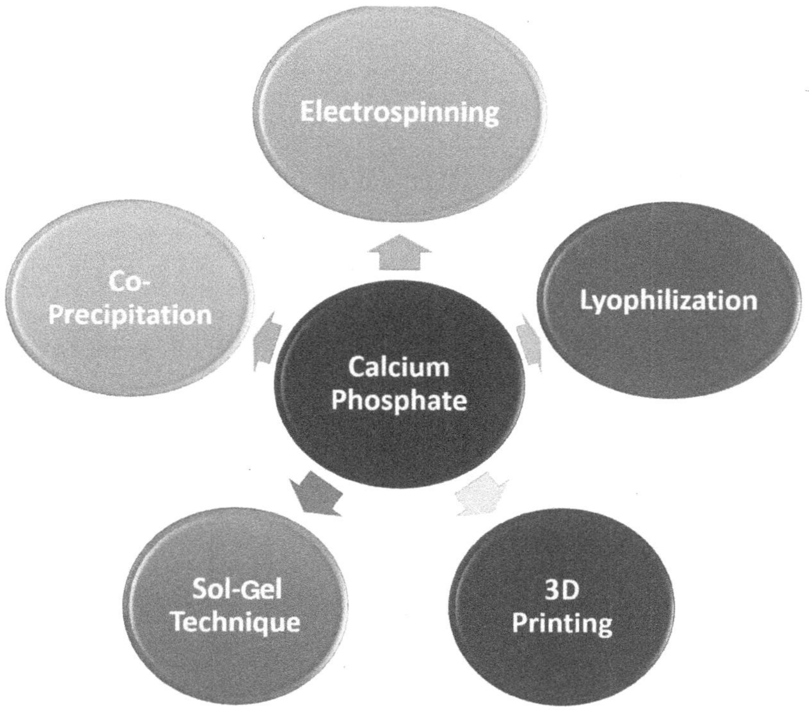

Figure 9.1 Diagrammatic representation of types of fabrication methods of calcium phosphate-based drug delivery systems.

phosphate-based drug delivery systems, ultimately enhancing their effectiveness in bone tissue engineering and regenerative medicine applications [30].

9.2.1 SOL-GEL METHOD

The sol-gel method is a versatile and widely used technique for the fabrication of various materials, including calcium phosphate-based drug delivery systems. It involves the conversion of a colloidal suspension (sol) into a 3D solid network (gel) through a series of chemical reactions [32]. In the context of calcium phosphate-based drug delivery systems, the sol-gel method allows for the controlled incorporation of drugs or bioactive molecules into the calcium phosphate matrix, providing a tailored drug release profile for bone tissue engineering applications [33]. The sol-gel process typically starts with the preparation of a sol, which consists of a dispersion of nanoparticles, usually calcium and phosphate precursors, in a liquid medium, often water or alcohol [34]. The drug or bioactive agent is then added to the sol, leading to the adsorption or chemical binding of the drug molecules onto the nanoparticle surfaces. The drug-incorporated sol is then allowed to undergo hydrolysis and condensation reactions, which promote the formation of a gel network [35, 36]. These reactions

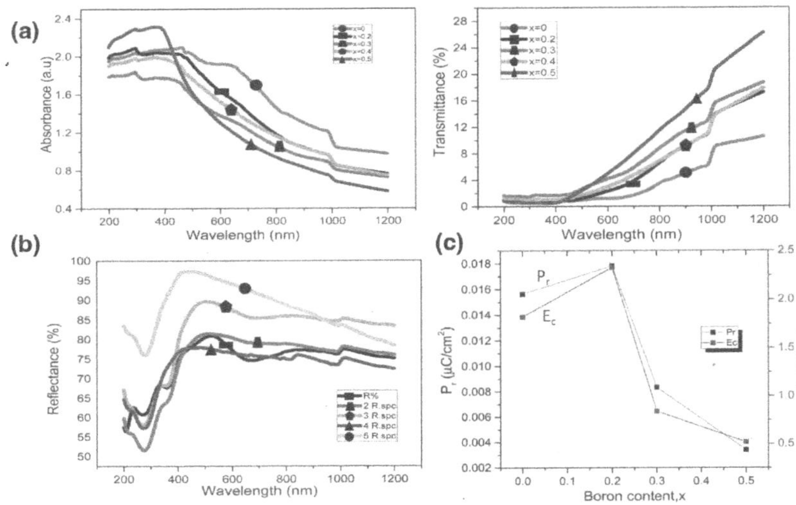

Figure 9.2 UV-shielding properties such as (a) Absorbance, Transmittance. (b) Reflectance. (c) P_r and E_C vs. Boron content describing ferroelectric properties [31]. (Reprinted from Al Hammad *et al.* Copyrights Elsevier 2016.)

result in the creation of a porous, interconnected structure that entraps the drug within the calcium phosphate matrix.

AlHammad et al. [31] synthesized nanostructured boron doped hydroxyapatite nanopowders using sol-gel technique. The UV-shielding and electrical properties of the prepared samples were investigated for drug-delivery applications. The results exhibited the good UV-shielding property in UV region and ceramics also indicated ferroelectric behavior as shown in Figure 9.2(a–c). It was concluded that boron doped hydroxyapatite exhibits the good drug delivery capability.

The sol-gel technique offers several advantages, including the ability to produce materials with precisely controlled composition, morphology, and porosity. It also allows the incorporation of dopants and other additives during the synthesis process. The method is particularly useful for creating thin films, coatings, and nanostructures, making it highly valuable in various applications, including optics, electronics, catalysis, and biomedical materials such as bioactive glasses used in bone tissue engineering.

9.2.2 ELECTROSPINNING

The electrospinning technique is a versatile and widely used method for fabricating nanofibers from various materials, including polymers, ceramics, and composites [37]. In the context of calcium phosphate-based drug delivery systems for bone tissue engineering, electrospinning allows for the creation of nanofibrous scaffolds with high surface area and controlled drug release properties [38]. The electrospinning process involves the application of an electric field to a polymer solution or melt, forcing the material to form a thin jet of fluid. As the jet travels toward a grounded collector, it undergoes elongation and whipping due to the electrostatic forces [39]. During this process, solvent evaporation occurs, leading to the solidification of the polymer into ultrafine fibers with diameters ranging from tens of nanometers to a few micrometers. To fabricate calcium phosphate-based drug delivery systems, calcium phosphate nanoparticles and the drug are incorporated into the polymer solution before electrospinning [40]. The nanoparticles and drug molecules become distributed within the polymer matrix, ensuring uniform drug loading throughout the nanofibers. By adjusting the concentration of calcium phosphate nanoparticles and the drug in the polymer solution, researchers can precisely control the drug release rate and overall drug delivery profile [41].

Fu et al. [42] synthesized amorphous calcium phosphate(ACP) nanoparticles and ACP-PLA nanofibres using electrospinning technique. As PLA is water soluble drug and these water soluble drugs are incompatible with electrospin technique, so lecithin is used as a surfactant for compatibility. The prepared samples revealed fast mineralization and drug release behavior in simulated body fluid. It was concluded that high biocompatibility, drug-release capacity and fast mineralization property revealed high potential application in tissue engineering.

Moreover, the electrospinning process is adaptable and allows for the incorporation of functional additives, nanoparticles, or bioactive molecules into the nanofibers, enhancing their properties and expanding their potential applications. While electrospinning has proven to be a versatile technique, challenges still exist, such as scalability and process control. However, ongoing research and development in this field are continually improving electrospinning methods, making it an increasingly important tool for nanomaterials fabrication and numerous advanced applications.

9.3 THERAPEUTIC AGENTS FOR BONE TISSUE ENGINEERING

Therapeutic agents used in bone tissue engineering aim to promote bone regeneration, enhance tissue healing, and prevent or treat complications associated with bone defects and fractures [43]. These agents can be categorized into several groups based on their specific functions. These agents encompass a combination of growth factors and antimicrobial agents, synergistically working together to address two key challenges in the field [44]. The combination of growth factors and antimicrobial agents in bone tissue engineering not only facilitates the repair of bone defects but also enhances the overall success and longevity of the implanted constructs, offering a promising approach to address various skeletal disorders and traumatic injuries [45].

9.3.1 GROWTH FACTORS

Growth factors are a group of essential signaling proteins that play fundamental roles in regulating cell growth, proliferation, and differentiation. These bioactive molecules are produced by various cells within the body and act as messengers to transmit important signals from one cell to another [46]. In the context of tissue engineering, growth factors are particularly vital for stimulating and guiding the regeneration and repair of damaged or injured tissues. Different types of growth factors, such as bone morphogenetic proteins (BMPs), platelet-derived growth factors (PDGFs), fibroblast growth factors (FGFs), insulin-like growth factors (IGFs), and vascular endothelial growth factors (VEGFs), among others, are utilized to trigger specific cellular responses [47–49]. Each growth factor has unique functions, influencing cellular behavior, tissue formation, and vascularization.

Incorporating growth factors into bone tissue engineering scaffolds, implants, or delivery systems allows for controlled and localized release, optimizing their therapeutic effects. This targeted approach minimizes potential side effects and systemic exposure while maximizing their impact on bone regeneration [50]. Growth factors have demonstrated their potential to significantly enhance bone healing in preclinical and clinical studies. They are particularly valuable in complex bone fractures, non-union fractures, and critical-size bone defects, where conventional treatments may be less effective [51]. However, challenges remain in precisely controlling their release kinetics, maintaining their stability, and managing potential immune responses. Future research is likely to focus on fine-tuning growth factor delivery systems and combining them with other therapeutic agents, such as antimicrobial agents, to achieve more robust and efficient bone tissue engineering strategies.

9.3.2 ANTIMICROBIAL AGENTS

Antimicrobial agents serve as valuable therapeutic agents to address the dual challenges of promoting bone regeneration while preventing and managing infections. Bone tissue engineering often involves the use of biomaterials and growth factors to stimulate bone healing and regeneration [54]. However, implant-associated infections can hinder the success of these approaches. By incorporating antimicrobial agents into the bone tissue engineering constructs, such as using antibiotic-loaded scaffolds or coatings, the risk of infection can be significantly reduced [55]. These agents help to combat and control bacterial colonization at the implant site, safeguarding the newly formed bone and promoting a favorable environment for bone regeneration.

Reibeiro et al. [52] synthesized gentamicin sulphate (GS) loaded calcium phosphate cements for drug delivery application. The liquid phase content and polymer type was changed in every sample for better efficiency. The results revealed that liquid phase content, i.e. (38%–42%) of calcium phosphate cement and use of hydroxypropyl methylcellulose (HPMC) polymer with 1.87% GS loading showed best formulation with suitable setting and mechanical properties as well as injectability. It also showed best antimicrobial activity against *S. epidermidis*, and *S. aureus* as shown in Figure 9.3(a). Song et al. [56] prepared cefazolin/chitosan, and cefazolin/chitosan cross-linked by calcium phosphate samples and then electrophoretically deposited on titanium. The results exhibited that cefazolin/chitosan samples showed better drug loading capacity but calcium phosphate cross-linked samples revealed better drug release capability. The samples showed good antimicrobial activity due to inclusion of cefazolin drug.

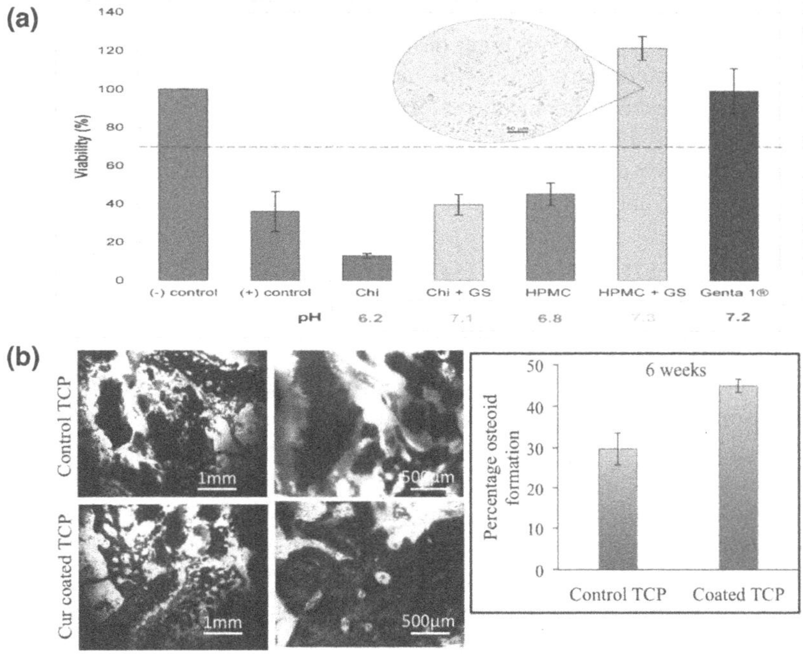

Figure 9.3 (a) MG63 cell viability after grown for 24 hour on different synthesized samples [52]. (Reprinted from Reibeiro *et al.* Copyrights Elsevier 2022.) (b) Optical microscopy images of tissue-implant sections showing new bone formation of uncoated and Curcumin coated tricalcium phosphate [53]. (Reprinted from Bose *et al.* Copyrights Elsevier 2018.)

The combination of antimicrobial agents with growth factors and biomaterials enhances the overall success and longevity of the implanted constructs, making it a promising strategy to address bone defects, fractures, and other skeletal disorders effectively. By effectively managing infections while supporting bone regeneration, antimicrobial agents play a crucial role in advancing the field of bone tissue engineering and improving patient outcomes.

9.4 DRUG DELIVERY INFLUENCE ON BONE REGENERATION

Drug delivery systems play a critical role in influencing bone regeneration when combined with calcium phosphate biomaterials. Calcium phosphate compounds, such as hydroxyapatite and tricalcium phosphate, are commonly used as scaffolds in bone tissue engineering due to their biocompatibility and osteoconductive properties [57]. When integrated with drug delivery systems, these biomaterials become powerful tools for promoting bone regeneration. Drug-loaded calcium phosphate scaffolds enable the controlled and localized release of growth factors, antimicrobial agents, and other therapeutic molecules directly to the defect site [58]. This targeted delivery enhances the recruitment and differentiation of bone-forming cells, accelerates the deposition of mineralized matrix, and fosters the integration of the scaffold with the surrounding bone tissue. Additionally, drug delivery systems in calcium phosphate constructs offer the advantage of sustained release, ensuring a prolonged and optimal therapeutic effect over time [59]. The combination of calcium phosphate and drug delivery technology represents a promising approach for successful bone tissue engineering, offering significant potential for treating bone defects, fractures, and skeletal disorders more effectively.

9.4.1 ENHANCED OSTEOGENESIS AND MINERALIZATION

Drug delivery systems can have a profound impact on bone regeneration by enhancing osteogenesis (the formation of new bone tissue) and mineralization (the deposition of minerals, such as calcium and phosphate, onto the bone matrix) [60]. By incorporating growth factors and other bioactive molecules within drug delivery systems, such as calcium phosphate scaffolds or implants, therapeutic agents can be precisely and locally delivered to the site of bone defects or injuries [61]. This targeted delivery stimulates the proliferation and differentiation of bone-forming cells, particularly osteoblasts, which are responsible for producing new bone tissue. Growth factors, like bone morphogenetic proteins (BMPs) or insulin-like growth factors (IGFs), promote the recruitment and differentiation of mesenchymal stem cells into osteoblasts, thereby accelerating the bone healing process [62,63]. Furthermore, drug delivery systems can sustain the release of these bioactive agents over time, ensuring a continuous and optimal concentration at the defect site, which is crucial for successful bone regeneration.

Bose et al. [53] studied release and effect of curcumin on hydroxyapatite coated titanium substrate. They used poly-caprolactone (PCL), poly ethylene glycol (PEG) and polylactide co glycolide (PLGA) as polymeric system to enhance drug release property. The results revealed that curcumin-PCL-PEG coated samples showed highest cell viability and complete mineralized bone formation as shown in Figure 9.3(b). It was concluded that synthesized samples can be regarded as excellent candidate for load bearing drug delivery applications. Zhou et al. [64] synthesized calcium phosphate-phosphorylated adenosine (CPPA) to study drug delivery applications for bone tissue engineering. The samples were synthesized using microwave assisted solvothermal technique. The samples showed high doxorubicin loading capacity and favorable osseointegration property for bone regeneration. The prepared samples displayed excellent drug delivery ability.

Furthermore, drug delivery systems can be customized to suit the specific needs of individual patients and the characteristics of their bone defects, allowing for personalized treatment approaches. This customization optimizes the therapeutic outcomes and minimizes potential complications, leading to improved patient satisfaction and quality of life. Overall, drug delivery systems have a remarkable impact on bone regeneration, enhancing osteogenesis and mineralization by providing controlled and targeted delivery of growth factors and essential minerals directly to the site of bone defects or injuries. As these technologies continue to advance, they hold tremendous promise for revolutionizing bone regeneration approaches and improving patient outcomes in the field of regenerative medicine.

9.4.2 PREVENTION OF INFECTION

The integration of drug delivery systems in bone regeneration plays a pivotal role in preventing infections and ensuring successful healing. During bone tissue engineering procedures, the use of implants or scaffolds can create a potential risk of bacterial colonization and infection, which can impede the regenerative process [66, 67]. Drug delivery systems offer a strategic solution by precisely delivering antimicrobial agents directly to the site of bone defects or implants. This localized delivery enables high concentrations of antimicrobial agents to combat bacteria effectively without causing systemic side effects [68]. The controlled and sustained release of these agents creates an antimicrobial environment around the implant, protecting it from potential infections during the critical phases of bone healing [69].

Sun et al. [65] studied 3D printed calcium phosphate scaffolds for antibacterial property. Calciumphosphate powders and berberine were used as printing inks. The concentration and cross-linking time of calcium chloride is adjusted to study efficiency of different prepared samples. The in-vitro biological tests revealed low cytotoxicity as shown in Figure 9.4(a–c) and sustained release of antimicrobial drugs, making it a promising candidate for drug delivery applications. Abkar et al. [70] studied the comparison between calcium phosphate, aluminium hydroxide and chitosan nanoparticles as drug delivery systems for immunization. The brucella melitensis was used to study the protection and immunization of different samples. The results revealed that samples containing calcium phosphate nanoparticles showed best results in terms of immunization and came out to be a potent antigen delivery systems.

These systems offer a targeted and efficient approach to maintain a sterile and conducive environment for bone healing, making them an essential component in advancing the field of bone tissue engineering and ensuring positive outcomes for patients undergoing bone regeneration therapies. As research in drug delivery technology progresses, there is great potential to further enhance infection prevention strategies in bone regeneration, promoting improved patient outcomes and better quality of life.

9.5 CONCLUSION AND FUTURE PERSPECTIVES

In conclusion, calcium phosphate-based biomaterials have emerged as promising platforms for drug delivery in bone tissue engineering. Their biocompatibility, osteoconductive properties, and resemblance to natural bone make them ideal candidates for supporting bone regeneration. By incorporating drug delivery systems into these biomaterials, therapeutic agents, including growth factors and antimicrobial agents, can be precisely and locally delivered to the site of bone defects or implants. This targeted and sustained delivery enhances osteogenesis, mineralization, and prevents infections, significantly improving the overall success and efficiency of bone regeneration procedures. The field of calcium phosphate-based biomaterials

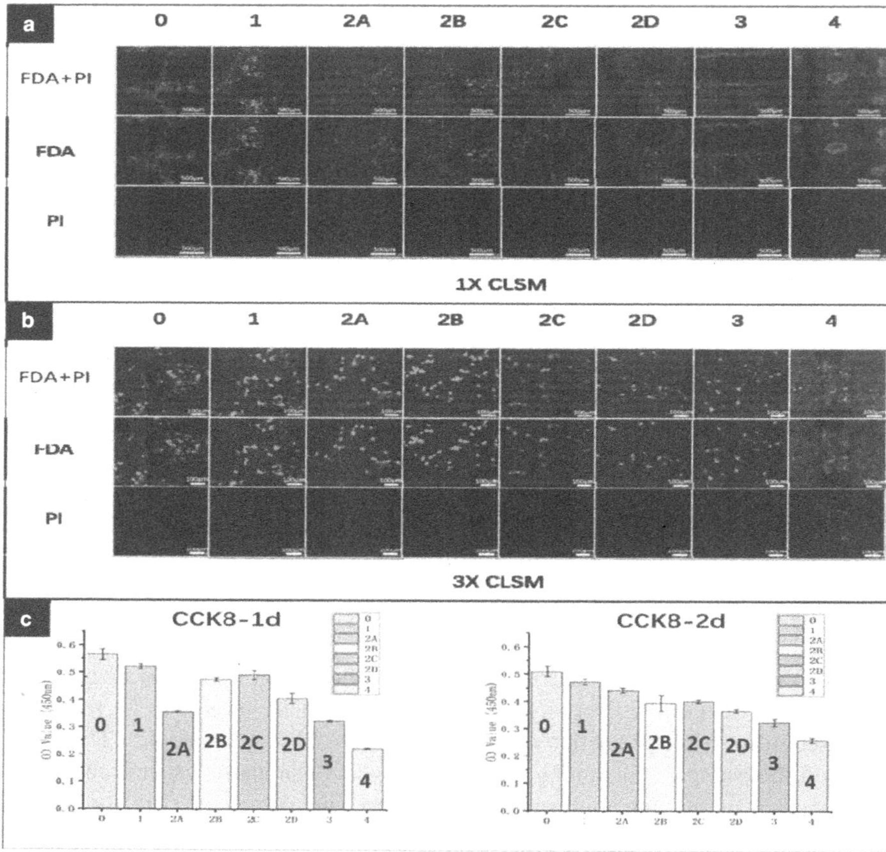

Figure 9.4 Cytotoxicity test results of the scaffolds, (a) Low magnification of FDA and PI staining results. (b) High magnification of FDA and PI staining results. (c) The results of CCK8 experiment on different synthesized samples [65]. (Reprinted from Sun *et al.* Copyrights Elsevier 2020.)

for drug delivery in bone tissue engineering is poised for continued growth and innovation. Researchers are likely to explore novel drug delivery strategies, such as advanced nanotechnology-based approaches, to further improve the controlled release of therapeutic agents. Additionally, the development of combination therapies, where multiple growth factors and antimicrobial agents are integrated into a single delivery system, may lead to even more robust and synergistic effects on bone regeneration and infection prevention. Furthermore, advancements in personalized medicine and tissue engineering techniques could enable the customization of drug delivery systems to match individual patient needs and specific bone defects. Tailoring drug release profiles and dosage to the patient's unique characteristics could optimize treatment outcomes and minimize potential complications. Moreover, ongoing efforts to improve the long-term stability and mechanical properties of calcium phosphate-based biomaterials will be crucial to ensure their successful integration with the surrounding bone tissue and to support the regenerative process over time. As researchers continue to explore new biomaterial formulations, drug combinations, and delivery approaches, the field of calcium phosphate-based drug delivery in bone tissue engineering holds great promise for addressing complex bone-related conditions, fractures, and skeletal disorders more effectively, ultimately leading to improved patient outcomes and quality of life.

REFERENCES

1. C. Xie, H. Lu, W. Li, F.-M. Chen, and Y.-M. Zhao. The use of calcium phosphatebased biomaterials in implant dentistry. *Journal of Materials Science: Materials in Medicine*, **23**:853–862, 2012.
2. X. Hou, L. Zhang, Z. Zhou, X. Luo, T. Wang, X. Zhao, B. Lu, F. Chen, and L. Zheng. Calcium phosphate-based biomaterials for bone repair. *Journal of Functional Biomaterials*, **13**(4):187, 2022.
3. S. Bose and S. Tarafder. Calcium phosphate ceramic systems in growth factor and drug delivery for bone tissue engineering: A review. *Acta Biomaterialia*, **8**(4):1401–1421, 2012.
4. F. Hajiali, S. Tajbakhsh, and A. Shojaei. Fabrication and properties of polycaprolactone composites containing calcium phosphate-based ceramics and bioactive glasses in bone tissue engineering: A review. *Polymer Reviews*, **58**(1):164–207, 2018.
5. S. Jin, X. Xia, J. Huang, C. Yuan, Y. Zuo, Y. Li, and J. Li. Recent advances in PLGA-based biomaterials for bone tissue regeneration. *Acta Biomaterialia*, **127**:56–79, 2021.
6. H. Xie, Z. Gu, Y. He, J. Xu, C. Xu, L. Li, and Q. Ye. Microenvironment construction of strontium–calcium-based biomaterials for bone tissue regeneration: The equilibrium effect of calcium to strontium. *Journal of Materials Chemistry B*, **6**(15):2332–2339, 2018.
7. P. Wang, L. Zhao, J. Liu, M. D. Weir, X. Zhou, and H. H. K. Xu. Bone tissue engineering via nanostructured calcium phosphate biomaterials and stem cells. *Bone Research*, **2**(1):1–13, 2014.
8. N. Beheshtizadeh, M. Azami, H. Abbasi, and A. Farzin. Applying extrusionbased 3D printing technique accelerates fabricating complex biphasic calcium phosphate-based scaffolds for bone tissue regeneration. *Journal of Advanced Research*, **40**:69–94, 2022.
9. I. Denry and L. T. Kuhn. Design and characterization of calcium phosphate ceramic scaffolds for bone tissue engineering. *Dental Materials*, **32**(1):43–53, 2016.
10. Q. Liu, W. F. Lu, and W. Zhai. Toward stronger robocast calcium phosphate scaffolds for bone tissue engineering: A mini-review and meta-analysis. *Biomaterials Advances*, **134**:112578, 2022.
11. S. Gautam, D. Bhatnagar, D. Bansal, H. Batra, and N. Goyal. Recent advancements in nanomaterials for biomedical implants. *Biomedical Engineering Advances*, **3**:100029, 2022.
12. S. Gautam, D. Bansal, D. Bhatnagar, C. Sharma, and N. Goyal. Synthesis of iron-based nanoparticles by chemical methods and their biomedical applications. In *Oxides for Medical Applications*, 167–195. Elsevier, 2023.
13. A. D. Bagde, A. M. Kuthe, S. Quazi, V. Gupta, S. Jaiswal, S. Jyothilal, N. Lande, and S. Nagdeve. State of the art technology for bone tissue engineering and drug delivery. *Irbm*, **40**(3):133–144, 2019.

14. A. H. Choi and B. Ben-Nissan. Calcium phosphate nanocoatings and nanocomposites, part I: Recent developments and advancements in tissue engineering and bioimaging. *Nanomedicine*, **10**(14):2249–2261, 2015.
15. D. Bhatnagar, S. Gautam, H. Batra, and N. Goyal. Enhancement of fracture toughness in carbonate doped hydroxyapatite based nanocomposites: Rietveld analysis and mechanical behaviour. *Journal of the Mechanical Behavior of Biomedical Materials*, **142**:105814, 2023.
16. K. Thanigai Arul, E. Manikandan, and R. Ladchumananandasivam. Polymer-based calcium phosphate scaffolds for tissue engineering applications. In *Nanoarchitectonics in Biomedicine*, 585–618. Elsevier, 2019.
17. M. Tavoni, M. Dapporto, Anna Tampieri, and S. Sprio. Bioactive calcium phosphate-based composites for bone regeneration. *Journal of Composites Science*, **5**(9):227, 2021.
18. C. Sharma, D. Bansal, D. Bhatnagar, S. Gautam, and N. Goyal. Advanced nanomaterials: From properties and perspective applications to their interlinked confronts. In *Advanced Functional Nanoparticles "Boon or Bane" for Environment Remediation Applications: Combating Environmental Issues*, 1–6. Springer, 2023.
19. T. S. S. Carvalho, N. Ribeiro, P. M. C. Torres, J. C. Almeida, J. H. Belo, J. P. Araújo, A. Ramos, M. Oliveira, and S. M. Olhero. Magnetic polylactic acid-calcium phosphate-based biocomposite as a potential biomaterial for tissue engineering applications. *Materials Chemistry and Physics*, **296**:127175, 2023.
20. A. Salama. Recent progress in preparation and applications of chitosan/calcium phosphate composite materials. *International Journal of Biological Macromolecules*, **178**:240–252, 2021.
21. D. Bansal, D. Bhatnagar, D. Rana, and S. Gautam. Ferrite nanoparticles in food technology. In *Applications of Nanostructured Ferrites*, 295–314. Elsevier, 2023.
22. R. A. Surmenev and M. A. Surmeneva. A critical review of decades of research on calcium phosphate–based coatings: How far are we from their widespread clinical application? *Current Opinion in Biomedical Engineering*, **10**:35–44, 2019.
23. S. Gautam, J. Singhal, H. K. Lee, and K. H. Chae. Drug delivery of paracetamol by metal-organic frameworks (HKUST-1): Improvised synthesis and investigations. *Materials Today Chemistry*, **23**:100647, 2022.
24. Y. Xia, H. Chen, Y. Zhao, F. Zhang, X. Li, L. Wang, M. D. Weir, J. Ma, M. A. Reynolds, N. Gu, H. H. K. Xu. Novel magnetic calcium phosphatestem cell construct with magnetic field enhances osteogenic differentiation and bone tissue engineering. *Materials Science and Engineering: C*, **98**:30–41, 2019.
25. S. Gautam, V. Thakur, and N. Goyal. Nanoferrites as drug carriers in targeted drug delivery applications. In *Applications of Nanostructured Ferrites*, 161–178. Elsevier, 2023.
26. M.-H. Hong, J. H. Lee, H. S. Jung, H. Shin, and H. Shin. Biomineralization of bone tissue: Calcium phosphate-based inorganics in collagen fibrillar organic matrices. *Biomaterials Research*, **26**(1):42, 2022.
27. C. C. Rey, C. Combes, and C. Drouet. Synthesis and physical chemical characterizations of octacalcium phosphate–based biomaterials for hard-tissue regeneration. In *Octacalcium Phosphate Biomaterials*, 177–212. Elsevier, 2020.
28. A. Diez-Escudero, M. Espanol, and M.-P. Ginebra. Synthetic bone graft substitutes: Calcium-based biomaterials. In *Dental Implants and Bone Grafts*, 125–157. Elsevier, 2020.

29. K. M. Zakir Hossain, U. Patel, A. R. Kennedy, L. Macri-Pellizzeri, V. Sottile, D. M. Grant, B. E. Scammell, and I. Ahmed. Porous calcium phosphate glass microspheres for orthobiologic applications. *Acta Biomaterialia*, **72**:396–406, 2018.
30. J. Kost, J. Huwyler, and M. Puchkov. Calcium phosphate microcapsules as multifunctional drug delivery devices. *Advanced Functional Materials*, **33**:2303333, 2023.
31. M. S. AlHammad. Nanostructure hydroxyapatite based ceramics by sol gel method. *Journal of Alloys and Compounds*, **661**:251–256, 2016.
32. K. Ishikawa, E. Garskaite, and A. Kareiva. Sol–gel synthesis of calcium phosphatebased biomaterials–a review of environmentally benign, simple, and effective synthesis routes. *Journal of Sol-Gel Science and Technology*, **94**:551–572, 2020.
33. M. Catauro, F. Papale, L. Sapio, and S. Naviglio. Biological influence of Ca/P ratio on calcium phosphate coatings by sol-gel processing. *Materials Science and Engineering: C*, **65**:188–193, 2016.
34. A. Gozalian, A. Behnamghader, M. Daliri, and A. Moshkforoush. Synthesis and thermal behavior of Mg-doped calcium phosphate nanopowders via the sol gel method. *Scientia Iranica*, **18**(6):1614–1622, 2011.
35. N. Jmal and J. Bouaziz. Synthesis, characterization and bioactivity of a calciumphosphate glass-ceramics obtained by the sol-gel processing method. *Materials Science and Engineering: C*, **71**:279–288, 2017.
36. M. Malakauskaite-Petruleviciene, Z. Stankeviciute, G. Niaura, E. Garskaite, A. Beganskiene, and A. Kareiva. Characterization of sol-gel processing of calcium phosphate thin films on silicon substrate by ftir spectroscopy. *Vibrational Spectroscopy*, **85**:16–21, 2016.
37. L. Dejob, B. Toury, S. Tadier, L. Gremillard, C. Gaillard, and V. Salles. Electrospinning of in situ synthesized silica-based and calcium phosphate bioceramics for applications in bone tissue engineering: A review. *Acta Biomaterialia*, **123**:123–153, 2021.
38. X. Niu, Z. Liu, F. Tian, S. Chen, L. Lei, T. Jiang, Q. Feng, and Y. Fan. Sustained delivery of calcium and orthophosphate ions from amorphous calcium phosphate and poly (L-lactic acid)-based electrospinning nanofibrous scaffold. *Scientific Reports*, **7**(1):45655, 2017.
39. H. Zhang, Q.-W. Fu, T.-W. Sun, F. Chen, C. Qi, J. Wu, Z.-Y. Cai, Q.-R. Qian, and Y.-J. Zhu. Amorphous calcium phosphate, hydroxyapatite and poly (D, L-lactic acid) composite nanofibers: Electrospinning preparation, mineralization and in vivo bone defect repair. *Colloids and Surfaces B: Biointerfaces*, **136**:27–36, 2015.
40. S. Chahal, F. S. J. Hussain, A. Kumar, M. M. Yusoff, and M. S. B. A. Rasad. Electrospun hydroxyethyl cellulose nanofibers functionalized with calcium phosphate coating for bone tissue engineering. *RSC Advances*, **5**(37):29497–29504, 2015.
41. S. Jin, J. Li, J. Wang, J. Jiang, Y. Zuo, Y. Li, and F. Yang. Electrospun silver ion-loaded calcium phosphate/chitosan antibacterial composite fibrous membranes for guided bone regeneration. *International Journal of Nanomedicine*, **13**:4591–4605, 2018.
42. Q.-W. Fu, Y.-P. Zi, W. Xu, R. Zhou, Z.-Y. Cai, W.-J. Zheng, F. Chen, and Q.-R. Qian. Electrospinning of calcium phosphate-poly (D, L-lactic acid) nanofibers for sustained release of water-soluble drug and fast mineralization. *International Journal of Nanomedicine*, **11**:5087–5097, 2016.
43. J. A. Jadlowiec, A. B. Celil, and J. O. Hollinger. Bone tissue engineering: Recent advances and promising therapeutic agents. *Expert Opinion on Biological Therapy*, **3**(3):409–423, 2003.

44. C. J. Kowalczewski and J. M. Saul. Biomaterials for the delivery of growth factors and other therapeutic agents in tissue engineering approaches to bone regeneration. *Frontiers in Pharmacology*, **9**:513, 2018.
45. C. Xu, M. Wang, W. Guo, W. Sun, and Y. Liu. Curcumin in osteosarcoma therapy: Combining with immunotherapy, chemotherapeutics, bone tissue engineering materials and potential synergism with photodynamic therapy. *Frontiers in Oncology*, **11**:672490, 2021.
46. Y. Liu, Y. Ma, J. Zhang, Y. Yuan, and J. Wang. Exosomes: A novel therapeutic agent for cartilage and bone tissue regeneration. *Dose-Response*, **17**(4):1559325819892702, 2019.
47. J. H. Lee. Injectable hydrogels delivering therapeutic agents for disease treatment and tissue engineering. *Biomaterials Research*, **22**(1):1–14, 2018.
48. T. U. Wani, R. S. Khan, A. H. Rather, M. A. Beigh, and F. A. Sheikh. Local dual delivery therapeutic strategies: Using biomaterials for advanced bone tissue regeneration. *Journal of Controlled Release*, **339**:143–155, 2021.
49. B. Al-Sowayan, F. Alammari, and A. Alshareeda. Preparing the bone tissue regeneration ground by exosomes: From diagnosis to therapy. *Molecules*, **25**(18):4205, 2020.
50. G. Gainza, S. Villullas, J. L. Pedraz, R. M. Hernandez, and M. Igartua. Advances in drug delivery systems (DDSs) to release growth factors for wound healing and skin regeneration. *Nanomedicine: Nanotechnology, Biology and Medicine*, **11**(6):1551–1573, 2015.
51. F. Canfarotta, L. Lezina, A. Guerreiro, J. Czulak, A. Petukhov, A. Daks, K. Smolinska-Kempisty, A. Poma, S. Piletsky, and N. A. Barlev. Specific drug delivery to cancer cells with double-imprinted nanoparticles against epidermal growth factor receptor. *Nano Letters*, **18**(8):4641–4646, 2018.
52. N. Ribeiro, M. Reis, L. Figueiredo, A. Pimenta, L. F. Santos, A. C. Branco, A. P. Alves de Matos, M. Salema-Oom, A. Almeida, M. F. C. Pereira, R. Colaço, and A. P. Serro. Improvement of a commercial calcium phosphate bone cement by means of drug delivery and increased injectability. *Ceramics International*, **48**(22):33361–33372, 2022.
53. S. Bose, N. Sarkar, and D. Banerjee. Effects of PCL, PEG and PLGA polymers on curcumin release from calcium phosphate matrix for in vitro and in vivo bone regeneration. *Materials Today Chemistry*, **8**:110–120, 2018.
54. F. Foroutan, J. McGuire, P. Gupta, A. Nikolaou, B. A. Kyffin, N. L. Kelly, J. V. Hanna, J. Gutierrez-Merino, J. C. Knowles, S.-Y. Baek, E. Velliou, and D. Carta. Antibacterial copper-doped calcium phosphate glasses for bone tissue regeneration. *ACS Biomaterials Science & Engineering*, **5**(11):6054–6062, 2019.
55. Y. Assal, Y. Mizuguchi, M. Mie, and E. Kobatake. Growth factor tethering to protein nanoparticles via coiled-coil formation for targeted drug delivery. *Bioconjugate Chemistry*, **26**(8):1672–1677, 2015.
56. T.-Y. Song, Y.-H. Wang, H.-W. Chien, C.-H. Ma, C.-L. Lee, and S.-F. Ou. Synthesis of cross-linked chitosan by calcium phosphate as long-term drug delivery coating with cytocompatibility. *Progress in Organic Coatings*, **173**:107162, 2022.
57. M. R. Newman and D. S. W. Benoit. Local and targeted drug delivery for bone regeneration. *Current Opinion in Biotechnology*, **40**:125–132, 2016.
58. K. Aoki and N. Saito. Biodegradable polymers as drug delivery systems for bone regeneration. *Pharmaceutics*, **12**(2):95, 2020.

59. M. Rama and U. Vijayalakshmi. Drug delivery system in bone biology: An evolving platform for bone regeneration and bone infection management. *Polymer Bulletin*, **80**:7341–7388, 2022.
60. E. O'Neill, G. Awale, L. Daneshmandi, O. Umerah, and K. W.-H. Lo. The roles of ions on bone regeneration. Drug Discovery Today, **23**(4):879–890, 2018.
61. J. Miszuk, Z. Liang, J. Hu, H. Sanyour, Z. Hong, H. Fong, and H. Sun. Elastic mineralized 3D electrospun PCL nanofibrous scaffold for drug release and bone tissue engineering. *ACS Applied Bio Materials*, **4**(4):3639–3648, 2021.
62. L. Zhu, D. Luo, and Y. Liu. Effect of the nano/microscale structure of biomaterial scaffolds on bone regeneration. *International Journal of Oral Science*, **12**(1):6, 2020.
63. Z. Gu, S. Wang, W. Weng, X. Chen, L. Cao, J. Wei, J.-W. Shin, and J. Su. Influences of doping mesoporous magnesium silicate on water absorption, drug release, degradability, apatite-mineralization and primary cells responses to calcium sulfate based bone cements. *Materials Science and Engineering: C*, **75**:620–628, 2017.
64. Z.-F. Zhou, T.-W. Sun, F. Chen, D.-Q. Zuo, H.-S. Wang, Y.-Q. Hua, Z.-D. Cai, and J. Tan. Calcium phosphate-phosphorylated adenosine hybrid microspheres for anti-osteosarcoma drug delivery and osteogenic differentiation. *Biomaterials*, **121**:1–14, 2017.
65. H. Sun, C. Hu, C. Zhou, L. Wu, J. Sun, X. Zhou, F. Xing, C. Long, Q. Kong, J. Liang, Y. Fan, and X. Zhang. 3D printing of calcium phosphate scaffolds with controlled release of antibacterial functions for jaw bone repair. *Materials & Design*, **189**:108540, 2020.
66. R. Dorati, A. DeTrizio, T. Modena, B. Conti, F. Benazzo, G. Gastaldi, and I. Genta. Biodegradable scaffolds for bone regeneration combined with drug-delivery systems in osteomyelitis therapy. *Pharmaceuticals*, **10**(4):96, 2017.
67. S. Bose, N. Sarkar, and D. Banerjee. Natural medicine delivery from biomedical devices to treat bone disorders: A review. *Acta Biomaterialia*, **126**:63–91, 2021.
68. P. Makvandi, U. Josic, M. Delfi, F. Pinelli, V. Jahed, E. Kaya, M. Ashrafizadeh, A. Zarepour, F. Rossi, A. Zarrabi, T. Agarwal, E. N. Zare, M. Ghomi, T. K. Maiti, L. Breschi, and F. R. Tay. Drug delivery (nano)platforms for oral and dental applications: Tissue regeneration, infection control, and cancer management. *Advanced Science*, **8**(8):2004014, 2021.
69. M. Mulazzi, E. Campodoni, G. Bassi, M. Montesi, S. Panseri, F. Bonvicini, G. A. Gentilomi, A. Tampieri, and M. Sandri. Medicated hydroxyapatite/collagen hybrid scaffolds for bone regeneration and local antimicrobial therapy to prevent bone infections. *Pharmaceutics*, **13**(7):1090, 2021.
70. M. Abkar, S. Alamian, and N. Sattarahmady. A comparison between adjuvant and delivering functions of calcium phosphate, aluminum hydroxide and chitosan nanoparticles, using a model protein of brucella melitensis Omp31. *Immunology Letters*, **207**:28–35, 2019.

10 Biodiesel Production Using CaO-Based Heterogeneous Catalysts

Preparation and Performance Evaluation

Kamaldeep Singh Nigha and Shifa Naaz
Dr. S.S. Bhatnagar University Institute of Chemical Engineering and Technology, Panjab University, Chandigarh, India

Amrit Pal Toor
Dr. S.S. Bhatnagar University Institute of Chemical Engineering and Technology and Energy Research Centre, Panjab University, Chandigarh, India

10.1 INTRODUCTION

Biodiesel is a sustainable and replaceable, liquid fuel addressing the robust demand for alternative fuel in an era where fossil reserves are about to extinct by the end of the decade [4]. Biodiesel may be used directly in current diesel engines by modifying them slightly or in mixes with fossil fuel [1]. Additionally, biodiesel-fueled engines show a massive reduction in toxic emissions like NO_x SO_x, unburned hydrocarbons, and soot particles [10]. Recently, the selectivity for heterogeneous catalysts for biodiesel production has increased because they are easier to separate and extremely reusable compared to homogenous catalysts.

Trans-esterification a reaction of vegetable or animal oils with alcohol (ethanol or methanol) is the most potential process catalyzed by the basic catalysts for sustainable biodiesel production as shown in Figure 10.1. The conventional method to carry out the transesterification is based on using base catalysts such as NaOH, KOH, or $NaOCH_3$ [17]. However, commercial biodiesel production remained a vital topic among various researchers globally for one and half decades [16]. Soybean oil was transesterified in the presence of alumina-supported potassium. Perhaps the employment of homogeneous catalysts remained a prominent trend among manufacturers for biodiesel production. The washing of homogeneous catalysts requires a

DOI: 10.1201/9781003360605-10

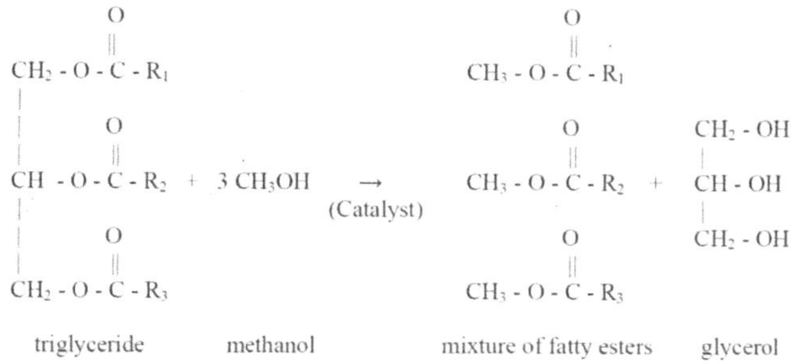

Figure 10.1 Transesterification reaction catalyzed by basic catalyst [69]. (Adapted from Ferreira et al. Copyrights Elsevier 2019.)

substantial quantity of freshwater, resulting in the formation of vast amounts of industrial effluent, making the process very environmentally detrimental. Therefore, heterogeneous catalysts can be a smart choice to reduce wastewater generation and cut the cost and energy usage by bypassing the unit operations involving catalyst separation.

Calcium oxides, which are ubiquitous in nature, are potential resources for the synthesis of heterogeneous catalysts for biodiesel generation via the transesterification process. Many .advances were demonstrated by many researchers employing calcium oxide-based catalysts to create biodiesels using pure, supported, and mixed metal oxides. However, the given material concentrates on calcium oxide derivatization and using it as a solid base catalyst for transesterification for prospective biodiesel yields from the standpoint of economic benefit [6]. CaO synthesis is far more convenient than that of many other solid catalysts, and the catalyst's catalytic activity may be increased by using thermal calcination. In the manufacture of CaO catalysts, several precursor salts such as carbonate, hydroxide, oxalate, and acetate monohydrate are used.

Table 10.1 compares both the advantages and disadvantages of several heterogeneous catalysts used in biodiesel generation. Calcium oxide is noted for its high activity and selectivity, making it an effective catalyst for this application, despite its limitations in non-basic reactions and its reactivity with water and acids. Other catalysts, such as zirconia, have high thermal and mechanical stability, while heteropolyacids and solid acid catalysts offer high activity and selectivity and can be reused. Montmorillonite, although limited in activity and selectivity, is abundant and low cost [7–9]. According to the study, calcium oxide is a highly potential catalyst for biodiesel synthesis due to its excellent selectivity, low cost, and ease of recovery. Calcium oxide has a low selectivity for non-basic reactions, which helps to prevent any unwanted side reactions. This makes it an ideal choice as a catalyst for the biodiesel production process.

Metal oxide nanoparticles have several uses in a variety of industries. Thereby, the synthesis of calcium oxide nanoparticles is attaining more attention among scientists because of its robust and better performance due to improved surface area

Table 10.1
Advantages and Disadvantages of Heterogeneous Catalysts for Biodiesel Production

Catalyst	Advantages	Disadvantages
Calcium oxide	• Demonstrates high activity and selectivity	• Limited utility in non-basic reactions
	• Efficiently eliminates side reactions	• Requires cautious handling due to its reactivity with water and acids
Zirconia	• Exhibits high thermal and mechanical stability	• Limited activity and selectivity
	• Suitable for continuous operation	• Can be relatively expensive
Heteropolyacids	• Demonstrates high activity and selectivity	• Can be relatively expensive
	• Capable of being reused	
Solid acid catalysts	• Demonstrates high activity and selectivity	• Limited stability under high temperatures
	• Capable of being reused	
Montmorillonite	• Abundant and cost-effective	• Limited activity and selectivity

[14]. The major challenge for calcium oxide synthesis is the selection of the source from which the Calcium oxide can potentially be synthesised.Various sources from which calcium oxide can be obtained include seashells, eggshells, bones, construction waste, oyster shells, dolomite rock, etc. Calcium oxide can be extracted from pulverized limestone and calcium chloride at high temperatures and pressure. Another method to derive calcium oxide is by electrolysis of calcium chloride solution.

Calcium oxide catalyst characteristics and catalytic activity are affected by a variety of parameters, including production process, calcination temperature, and surface area. Furthermore, X-ray diffraction, scanning electron microscopy, transmission electron microscopy, Fourier-transform infrared spectroscopy, and BET surface area analysis are commonly used in the characterisation of CaO catalysts [15]. X-ray diffraction can indicate the crystalline phases present in the catalyst, whilst microscopy can reveal its shape and particle size [18]. The catalyst's surface functional groups and chemical makeup may be determined using Fourier-transform infrared spectroscopy, and its surface area and pore size distribution can be determined using BET surface area analysis [11]. Understanding the composition and characteristics of CaO catalysts with the use of these characterisation approaches can help to improve the catalysts' efficiency in a variety of catalytic processes.

By transesterifying lipid oils with short-chain alcohols like methanol, ethanol, or propanol, which are a plentiful supply of triglycerides, diglycerides, and monoglycerides, biodiesel may be produced. However, high levels of free fatty acids (FFAs) in these oils can cause saponification, a side reaction that can limit the efficiency of the process [5]. As shown in Figure 10.2, to prevent saponification, esterification of the oil is carried out as a pre-treatment step using an acid catalyst such as H_2SO_4, HCl, or heterogeneous catalysts. This step converts FFAs to esters that do not interfere with the transesterification reaction [12]. Therefore, it is crucial to carefully select the raw materials, ensuring that the oil has low levels of FFAs or that proper pretreatment is carried out to avoid the formation of side products [2]. Studies have shown that the presence of FFAs can significantly affect the biodiesel yield and quality. Proper pretreatment of high FFA oils can lead to improved biodiesel yield and quality [13]. In addition, several studies have investigated the use of different catalysts for esterification, including homogeneous and heterogeneous catalysts [3]. Overall, careful consideration of the raw materials and appropriate pretreatment steps, including esterification, can ensure efficient and high-quality biodiesel production.

In addition, a transesterification process can be accomplished using the catalyst. As a result, while talking about the transesterification of calcium oxide as a heterogeneous base to produce biodiesel, reaction optimisation becomes a crucial factor that

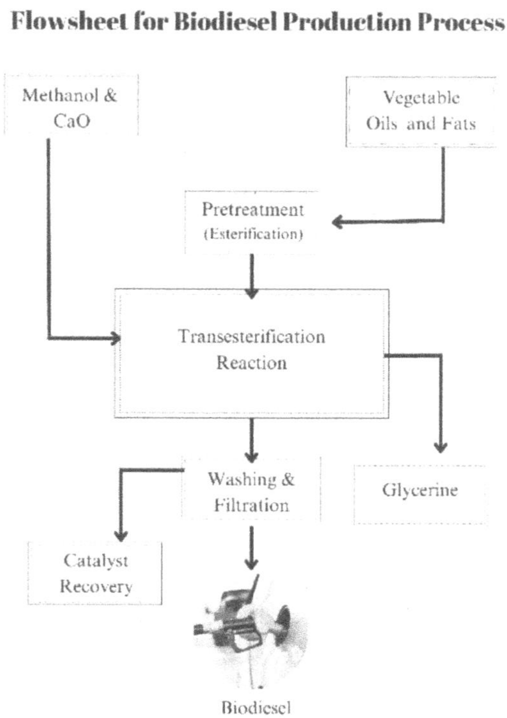

Figure 10.2 Flowsheet of biodiesel production.

must be taken into account. Temperature, the amount of catalyst used, the alcohol-to-oil molar ratio, and the reaction duration are the main factors impacting the rates of the transesterification reaction and the FAME conversion. Additionally, a number of particular factors should be considered, including FFA, water content, the usage of a support for the catalyst, total basic sites, calcination temperature, and reusability of the catalyst.

10.2 METHODOLOGY

Calcium oxide has been identified as a highly promising catalyst for sustainable applications due to its strong basic properties and ability to tolerate high levels of free fatty acids, making it a potential catalyst for transesterification reactions [19]. Additionally, calcium oxide has low solubility in methanol, leading to high catalyst recovery rates [20]. This results in a catalyst with a large pore diameter and high surface area, which is essential for the diffusion of reactants on the catalyst surface [21]. Another method for obtaining calcium oxide involves electrolysis of calcium chloride solution [22].

10.2.1 SOURCES TO DERIVE CALCIUM OXIDE

Calcium oxide can be derived from various sources such as seashells, eggshells, bones, construction waste, oyster shells, dolomite rock, etc. [23, 24] (Figure 10.3). The yield of product obtained from calcium oxide sources depends upon feedstock and the source of calcium oxide catalyst derivation [25]. While not naturally occurring, calcium oxide can be obtained from pulverized limestone and calcium chloride through the process of calcination at high temperatures and pressures, typically between 800 and 1300°C [26]. Another way to produce calcium oxide is through the

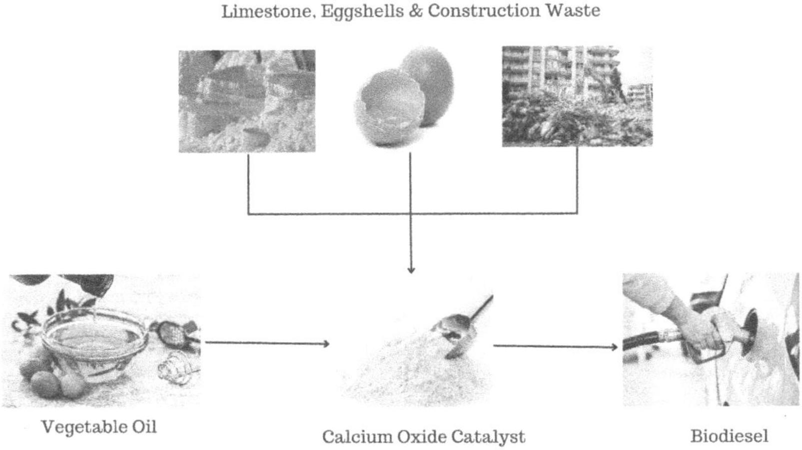

Figure 10.3 Pictorial representation to various sources of calcium oxide catalyst.

electrolysis of calcium chloride solution [27]. These methods are commonly used in industrial processes to obtain calcium oxide for various applications.

10.2.1.1 Calcium Oxide Catalyst Derived from the Eggshell

Eggshells can serve as a sustainable source of calcium oxide, which can be used in various industries such as catalysts, construction materials, and wastewater treatment. The process of eggshell to calcium oxide conversion includes multiple steps such as washing, drying, grinding, acid treatment, and calcination [28]. Eggshells are washed repeatedly to remove impurities, dirt, and interfering materials. The eggshells are pulverised using ball mills into a uniform 40 μm powder after drying for 24 hours at 100°C in an oven. A mild acid is used to dissolve the calcium carbonate in the eggshell, resulting in the production of calcium acetate and carbon dioxide gas. The resulting material is then calcined in a muffle furnace at high temperatures of 800–900°C to produce calcium oxide nanoparticles. The utilization of eggshells as a raw material can reduce the need for traditional sources of calcium oxide, such as limestone, which leads to environmental degradation due to mining and processing. This technique provides a sustainable source of raw material for various industries [29]. The calcium oxide nanoparticles obtained have a high surface area and reactivity, making them useful in different applications.

10.2.1.2 Calcium Oxide Catalyst Derived from Seashell

Seashells are considered waste material, but they can be utilized in calcium oxide catalyst preparation. There are various types of seashells available such as oyster shells, mussel shells, scallop shells, periwinkle shells, and cockle shells [30]. Different types of seashells produce different yields of calcium oxide catalysts. The shells are calcined at 700–1000°C in an air atmosphere for 4 h, the calcium carbonate is dissociated to form calcium oxide [31]. The resulting solid formed is then crushed and subjected to pass through 100–200 mesh [31]. The resulting product obtained contains particles of 38–75 μm [31].

10.2.1.3 Calcium Oxide Catalyst Derived from Construction Waste

The construction sites, industries, and households produce a significant amount of waste daily which is normally dumped in landfills or left on the sites due to inadequate management and a lack of waste utilization techniques [32]. The construction waste contains materials like cement, concrete, gypsum, and bricks which are viable sources to derive calcium oxide. The methodologies involved proves to be a viable technology to produce catalyst along with addressing the complete utilization to reuse and regenerate effective calcium oxide catalyst from construction waste [34]. This waste collected from various demolition sites is first screened to remove unnecessary particles. Then further the raw material is grounded into finer particles and then calcination at 700°C is done which gives us are required product that calcium oxide catalyst that can be further used for catalytic applications such as pyrolysis, gasification, and majorly biodiesel production [33].

10.2.1.4 Calcium Oxide Catalyst Derived from Pulverized Limestone

Calcium oxide is also derived from pulverized limestone through a process called calcination [35]. This involves heating the limestone to temperatures between 800°C and 1300°C, which causes it to decompose and release carbon dioxide, leaving behind calcium oxide. The resulting product is a white, powdery substance with strong basic properties that make it useful for various industrial applications, including the production of biodiesel along with cement, steel, and chemicals [35]. The calcination process has been extensively studied and is well-documented in the literature, with several studies examining the effects of calcination temperature, duration, and feedstock composition on the quality and properties of the resulting calcium oxide [22, 36].

10.2.2 DOPING OF CALCIUM OXIDE CATALYST FOR BIODIESEL PRODUCTION

Agglomeration of pure species reduces catalytic efficiency; hence, calcium oxide is often doped with transition metals to increase the number of active sites. The catalytic efficiency of calcium oxide can be improved by a variety of doping techniques, including wetness impregnation, co-precipitation, and sol–gel procedures [38]. Several processes, including the manufacture of biodiesel, have benefited from the successful doping of transition metals including Zr, Cu, Fe, and Co onto calcium oxide catalysts [39, 40]. The efficiency and selectivity of calcium oxide catalysts may be improved using these doping techniques, making them more appropriate for use in industrial applications.

Table 10.2 and Figure 10.4, present a comparative study of various catalysts doped with different materials for the production of biodiesel. The doping methods include co-precipitation, precipitation, wetness impregnation, ball milling, and sol–gel. The study found that cobalt-doped CaO, CaO-La_2O_3, and zinc oxide doped CaO catalysts show higher yield percentages of 98%, 98.76%, and 97.6%, respectively. The reaction time for producing biodiesel ranges from 80 minutes to 480 minutes. The study found that the cobalt-doped CaO catalyst requires the shortest reaction time of 120 minutes while the silicon oxide-based calcium oxide catalyst requires the longest time of 480 minutes. The reaction temperature ranges from 55 to 160°C, and the catalyst loading ranges from 0.2% to 8%. The alumina doped CaO catalyst shows the highest catalyst loading of 8%, while the lithium doped CaO catalyst shows the lowest catalyst loading of 0.2%.

In conclusion, Table 10.2 provides useful information for selecting appropriate catalysts and doping methods for the production of biodiesel. The study suggests that cobalt-doped CaO and CaO-La_2O_3 catalysts are highly effective for producing biodiesel with high yields, while the alumina doped CaO catalyst requires a higher catalyst loading. It is important to consider the reaction time, temperature, and catalyst loading for optimizing the biodiesel production process. The results presented in Table 10.2 can aid in selecting the most efficient catalyst for the production of biodiesel, which can have a positive impact on the environment and contribute to sustainable energy production.

Table 10.2

Comparison of Different Catalysts CaO-Based Doped Catalysts on the Basis of Preparation Technique, Oil: Methanol Ratio, Yield, Reaction Temperature, and Reaction Time.

Catalyst	Doping Method	Oil : Alcohol Ratio	Yield (%)	Reaction Time (min)	Reaction Temperature	Catalyst Loading (wt%)	References
Zinc-doped CaO	Co-precipitation	1:9	89	80	55	6	[41]
Alumina-doped CaO	Precipitation	1:9	92.5	90	65	8	[42]
Potassium and chromium-doped CaO	Wetness Impregnation	-	85.6	360	-	-	[43]
Cobalt-doped CaO	Co-precipitation	-	98	120	60	1.5	[44]
Barium doped CaO	Thermal decomposition	1:6	88	180	65	3	[45]
Lithium doped CaO	Wet impregnation	1:14	90	180	60	0.2	[46]
Zinc oxide-doped CaO	Ball milling - powder mixture of $Ca(OH)_2$ and ZnO	1:10	97.6	240	60	2	[47]
Zeolite supported CaO	Microwave irradiation	1:9	95	180	65	3	[48]
Silicon oxide based calcium oxide	Sol gel	1:16	85.6	480	60	6	[49]
CaO/ Biochar	Wet impregnation method	1:12	96	360	65	3	[50]
CaO–NiO	Co-precipitation,	1:15	>80	360	65	5	[51]
CaO-La_2O_3	Co-precipitation method	1:25	98.76	180	160	3	[52]
CaMgO and CaZnO	Coprecipitation method	1:15	>80	360	65	4	[53]

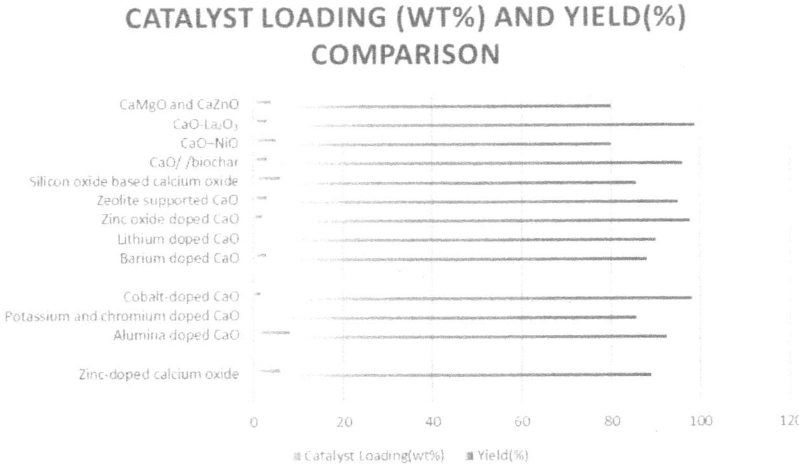

Figure 10.4 Graphical representation of catalyst loading and yield percentage for the different CaO-based doped catalysts.

10.3 MECHANISM OF TRANSESTERIFICATION REACTION WITH CALCIUM OXIDE

The process of producing biodiesel from triglycerides using CaO derived from waste eggshells is illustrated in Figure 10.5. The process initiates with the generation of a methoxide anion through the removal of an H^+ ion from the hydroxyl group of methanol by the O_2^- ion present on the catalyst surface. The methoxide anion, possessing alkaline properties, exhibits strong catalytic activity and plays a crucial role in the transesterification reaction. In the second step, a tetrahedral intermediate is formed when the methoxide anion attaches to the positively charged carbonyl carbon of the triglyceride molecules. Subsequently, in the third step, a tetrahedral intermediate acquires an H+ atom from the surface of calcium oxide. Finally, in the fourth step, the rearrangement of the tetrahedral intermediate leads to the formation of biodiesel (FAME). The reaction proceeds similarly for diglycerides and monoglycerides, resulting in the production of three moles of FAME and one mole of glycerol (as a by-product) for every mole of triglyceride.

10.4 MORPHOLOGY AND CHARACTERIZATION

The morphology of calcium oxide (CaO) is an important factor that affects its catalytic activity [55]. CaO can exist in various morphologies such as cubes, spheres, rods, and wires. The morphology of CaO is influenced by several factors such as the method of preparation, temperature, and pressure conditions during synthesis. Cubes are the most commonly observed morphology for CaO and are typically formed by the calcination of calcium carbonate [56]. Spheres and rods can be obtained through the precipitation method, where the morphology is controlled by the surfactant used

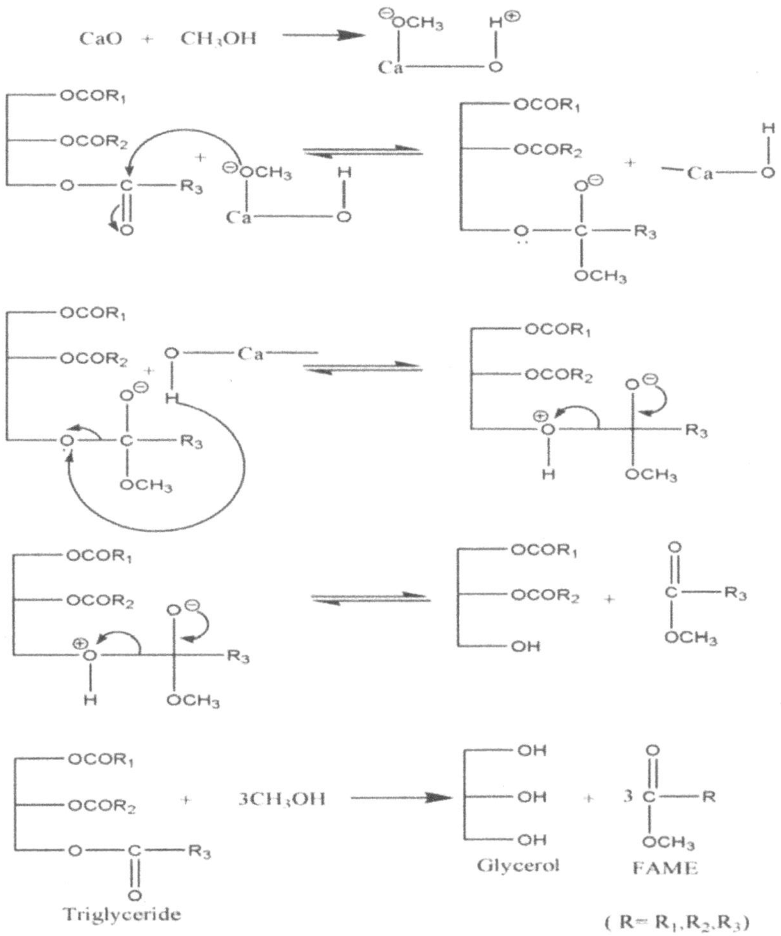

Figure 10.5 Mechanism of transesterification reaction with CaO catalyst.

during synthesis [53]. In recent years, nanoscale CaO particles have gained attention due to their high surface area and unique properties [54]. These nanoscale particles can be synthesized using various methods such as sol–gel, and hydrothermal methods. The synthesis of CaO nanoparticles with controlled morphology and size has led to improvements in catalytic activity in various applications. The morphology of CaO also plays a critical role in determining its surface area, pore volume, and pore size distribution, which are important factors in catalytic activity. For example, CaO nanoparticles with a higher surface area have been reported to exhibit superior catalytic activity in transesterification reactions compared to bulk CaO due to their higher surface area [52]. In summary, the morphology of CaO plays a significant role in determining its catalytic activity, and the control of morphology is a crucial step in the design of effective catalysts for various applications [51]. The morphology of calcium oxide-based catalysts can be controlled by the synthesis method, dopant concentration, and support materials. The morphology has a significant impact on the catalyst's performance in various applications, including biodiesel production, CO_2 capture, hydrogen production, and chemical synthesis. Nanocubes and nanosheets have been found to exhibit higher catalytic activity and stability compared to nanoparticles and microparticles due to their larger surface area and higher number of active sites (Figure 10.6).

XRD pattern of calcined eggshell at 900°C for 3 h was analyzed. The Joint Committee of Powder Diffracation Standards (JCPDS) database (00-37-1497) was used to compare the peaks. The intense peaks of calcined CaO at 2θ value, 32.69°, 37.63°, and 54.47° were detected. Different phases in calcined CaO were identified by their 2θ value (degree) [64] (Figure 10.7).

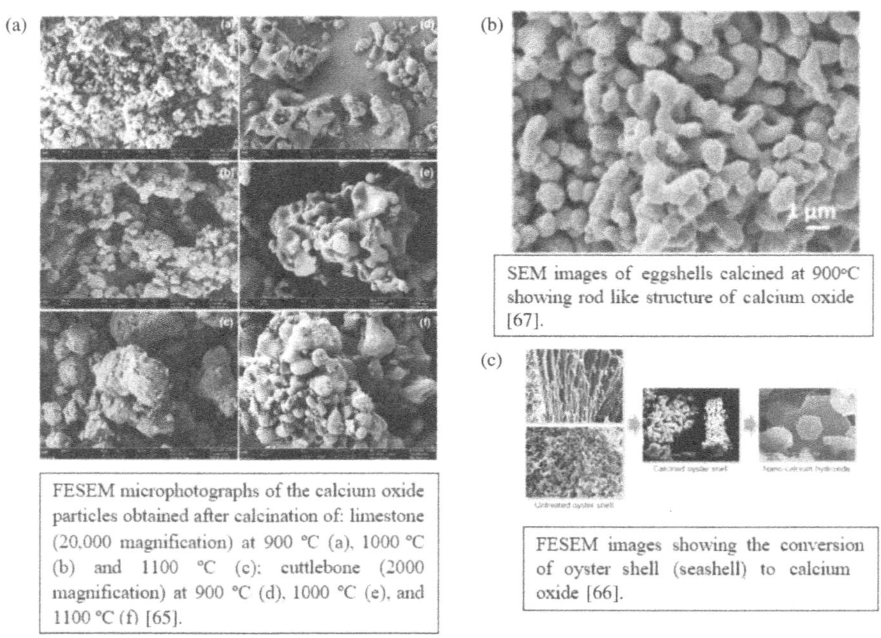

Figure 10.6 FESEM images of calcium oxide derived from different sources such as eggshells, seashells, limestone, etc. ((a) Copyright "Creative Commons Attribution 4.0 International" 2020 Consejo Superior de Investigaciones Científicas (CSIC). (b) Adapted from Kaou et al. Copyrights Wiley Online Library 2023. (c) Adapted from Mohd Danish Khan et al. Copyrights Elsevier 2018.)

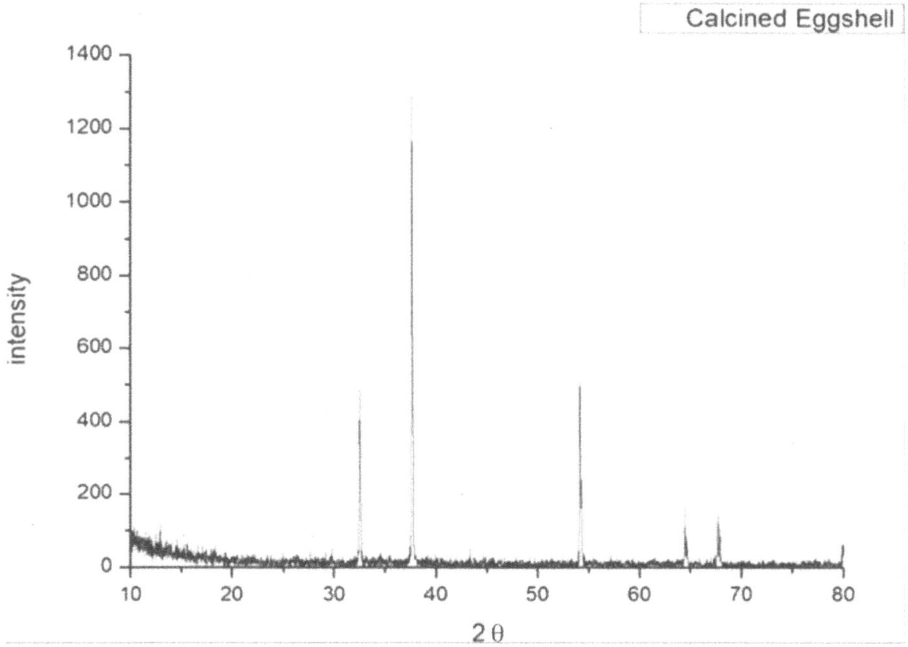

Figure 10.7 X-ray diffractogram of calcium oxide. Catalyst [64]. (Adapted from Bharti, et al. Copyrights Elsevier 2020.)

10.5 CONCLUSION

In conclusion, the utilization of calcium oxide (CaO) based catalysts for biodiesel production has emerged as a promising avenue in the quest for sustainable and environmentally friendly energy sources. The unique properties and numerous advantages of CaO catalysts have contributed to their increasing popularity in the field of biodiesel synthesis.

Firstly, CaO catalysts exhibit exceptional catalytic activity and stability, ensuring efficient and reliable biodiesel production. The high basicity of CaO enables it to effectively catalyze the transesterification reaction, facilitating the conversion of triglycerides into biodiesel. This characteristic contributes to cost reduction and enhances the economic viability of biodiesel production processes. Moreover, CaO catalysts offer several advantages from an environmental standpoint. Their production does not require expensive or hazardous materials, and the catalysts can be easily synthesized from abundant and inexpensive calcium-containing compounds. Furthermore, CaO is non-toxic and does not pose a threat to human health or the environment. This eco-friendly attribute aligns with the principles of sustainable development and supports the global efforts to mitigate climate change and reduce greenhouse gas emissions. The flexibility of CaO for wide range feedstocks enhances the feasibility of biodiesel production and allows for the utilization of diverse feedstock sources, including waste cooking oils and animal fats, thereby reducing waste and promoting a circular economy. In conclusion, the use of CaO oxide based catalysts in biodiesel production has shown great promise in terms of catalytic activity, stability, environmental friendliness, and feedstock versatility. As the demand for sustainable energy sources continues to grow, CaO catalysts offer a viable solution for the production of biodiesel on a large scale. Further research and development efforts should focus on optimizing the catalyst preparation methods, exploring catalyst regeneration techniques, and investigating the potential synergies with other catalysts or additives.

REFERENCES

1. Bukkarapu, K. R., & Krishnasamy, A. (2022). A critical review on available models to predict engine fuel properties of biodiesel. *Renewable and Sustainable Energy Reviews*, **155**, 111925. https://doi.org/10.1016/j.rser.2021.111925.
2. Demirbas, A. (2009). Progress and recent trends in biodiesel fuels. *Energy Conversion and Management*, **50**(1), 14–34. https://doi.org/10.1016/j.enconman.2008.09.001.
3. El-sherif, A. A., Hamad, A. M., Shams-Eldin, E., Mohamed, H. A. A. E., Ahmed, A. M., Mohamed, M. A., Abdelaziz, Y. S., Sayed, F. A.-Z., El qassem Mahmoud, E. A. A., Abd El-Daim, T. M., & Fahmy, H. M. (2023). Power of recycling waste cooking oil into biodiesel via green CaO-based eggshells/Ag heterogeneous nanocatalyst. *Renewable Energy*, **202**, 1412–1423. https://doi.org/10.1016/j.renene.2022.12.041.
4. Kalair, A., Abas, N., Saleem, M. S., Kalair, A. R., & Khan, N. (2021). Role of energy storage systems in energy transition from fossil fuels to renewables. *Energy Storage*, 3(1). https://doi.org/10.1002/est2.135.
5. Kokkinos, N., Theochari, G., Emmanouilidou, E., Angelova, D., Toteva, V., Lazaridou, A., & Mitkidou, S. (2022). Biodiesel production from high free fatty acid byproduct of bioethanol production process. *IOP Conference Series: Earth and Environmental Science*, **1123**(1), 012009. https://doi.org/10.1088/1755-1315/1123/1/012009.
6. Kouzu, M., Kasuno, T., Tajika, M., Sugimoto, Y., Yamanaka, S., & Hidaka, J. (2008). Calcium oxide as a solid base catalyst for transesterification of soybean oil and its application to biodiesel production. *Fuel*, **87**(12), 2798–2806. https://doi.org/10.1016/j.fuel.2007.10.019.
7. Maitra, S., & Sarkar, P. (2018). Review on characterization of solid catalysts for biodiesel production. *Energy Sources, Part A: Recovery, Utilization, and Environmental Effects*, **40**(19), 2333–2350.
8. Meher, L. C., Sagar, D. V., & Naik, S. N. (2006). Technical aspects of biodiesel production by transesterification—a review. *Renewable and Sustainable Energy Reviews*, **10**(3), 248–268. https://doi.org/10.1016/j.rser.2004.09.002.
9. Szymanowska-Powałowska, D., Kijeńska-Gawrońska, E., & Gryglewicz, G. (2021). Catalysts for the transesterification of vegetable oils: A review. *Catalysts*, **11**(4), 409. https://doi.org/10.3390/catal11040409.
10. Kulkarni, M. G., & Dalai, A. K. (2006). Waste cooking oil-an economical source for biodiesel: A review. *Industrial & Engineering Chemistry Research*, **45**(9), 2901–2913. https://doi.org/10.1021/ie0510526
11. Li, B., Hao, Y., Zhang, B., Shao, X., & Hu, L. (2017). A multifunctional noble-metal-free catalyst of CuO/TiO_2 hybrid nanofibers. *Applied Catalysis A: General*, **531**, 1–12. https://doi.org/10.1016/j.apcata.2016.12.002.

12. Marchetti, J. M., Miguel, V. U., & Errazu, A. F. (2007). Possible methods for biodiesel production. *Renewable and Sustainable Energy Reviews*, **11**(6), 1300–1311. https://doi.org/10.1016/j.rser.2005.08.006.
13. Noureddini, H., Gao, X., & Philkana, R. S. (2005). Immobilized *Pseudomonas cepacia* lipase for biodiesel fuel production from soybean oil. *Bioresource Technology*, **96**(7), 769–777. https://doi.org/10.1016/j.biortech.2004.05.029.
14. Oskam, G. (2006). Metal oxide nanoparticles: Synthesis, characterization and application. *Journal of Sol-Gel Science and Technology*, **37**(3), 161–164. https://doi.org/10.1007/s10971-005-6621-2.
15. Shylesh, S. (2006). Synthesis and characterization of organo modified metal containing mesoporous material for oxidation catalysis. In *Applied Chemistry and Chemical Engineering*, 3–28.
16. Xie, W., Peng, H., & Chen, L. (2006). Transesterification of soybean oil catalyzed by potassium loaded on alumina as a solid-base catalyst. *Applied Catalysis A: General*, **300**(1), 67–74. https://doi.org/10.1016/j.apcata.2005.10.048.
17. Yan, S., Kim, M., Salley, S. O., & Ng, K. Y. S. (2009). Oil transesterification over calcium oxides modified with lanthanum. *Applied Catalysis A: General*, **360**(2), 163–170. https://doi.org/10.1016/j.apcata.2009.03.015.
18. Yan, Z., Wang, Z., Liu, H., Tu, Y., Yang, W., Zeng, H., & Qiu, J. (2015). Decomposition and solid reactions of calcium sulfate doped with SiO_2, Fe_2O_3 and Al_2O_3. *Journal of Analytical and Applied Pyrolysis*, **113**, 491–498. https://doi.org/10.1016/j.jaap.2015.03.019.
19. Bhatia, R., & Sharma, Y. C. (2017). Advances in calcium oxide-based heterogeneous catalysts for biodiesel production. *Renewable and Sustainable Energy Reviews*, **69**, 558–579. https://doi.org/10.1016/j.rser.2016.11.140.
20. Kumar, P., & Sharma, Y. C. (2016). A review of recent advances in heterogeneous catalysts for biodiesel production. *Renewable and Sustainable Energy Reviews*, **55**, 249–282. https://doi.org/10.1016/j.rser.2015.10.006.
21. Chen, W., Wang, L., Liu, X., & Li, L. (2017). Preparation and characterization of calcium oxide catalysts for biodiesel production. *Energy Sources, Part A: Recovery, Utilization, and Environmental Effects*, **39**(15), 1591–1598.
22. Zhang, J., Chen, X., Li, J., Zhou, Y., & Cheng, J. (2018). Preparation of calcium oxide from waste eggshells by electrochemical synthesis. *Waste Management*, **74**, 70–75. https://doi.org/10.1016/j.wasman.2017.11.035.
23. Anjum, S., Raza, S. S., Khan, S., & Ali, A. (2022). production of calcium oxide from various sources: A review. *Chemical Engineering Transactions*, **90**, 97–102.
24. Viju, V. J., Raveendran, R., & Easo, J. G. (2022). A review on calcium oxide production from shells and waste eggshell management. *Journal of Cleaner Production*, **320**, 128819.
25. Sun, Y., Chen, Z., Wei, X., Zou, Y., Huang, L., & Zhou, M. (2021). Effects of different catalysts on thermal decomposition of dolomite for production of calcium oxide. *Journal of Thermal Analysis and Calorimetry*, **146**(1), 355–366.
26. Tian, Y., Li, D., Liu, J., Li, G., Li, Y., & Li, J. (2022). Facile and low-cost synthesis of hierarchical CaO from natural calcium carbonate for effective CO_2 capture. *Journal of Materials Science*, **57**(5), 3784–3794.
27. Zhang, S., Wei, X., Cai, Z., Jiang, J., & Wei, D. (2022). Facile synthesis of CaO microspheres for efficient CO_2 capture by the high-efficiency calcium looping process. *Journal of Environmental Management*, **306**, 114006.

28. Chen, Y., Huang, L., Xie, Z., & Wang, L. (2022). Calcium oxide nanoparticles derived from eggshells as a sustainable catalyst for biodiesel production. *Journal of Cleaner Production*, **319**, 128963.
29. Wang, Q., Zhang, Y., Wang, Z., Huang, X., Wang, M., & Zhang, J. (2021). Valorization of eggshell wastes to prepare calcium oxide nanoparticles and their application for efficient CO_2 capture. *Journal of Cleaner Production*, **297**, 126589.
30. Babatunde, O. M., Zhao, C., Chen, Z., Xie, X., & Niu, X. (2021). Characterization and application of seashell as a catalyst in biodiesel production. *Energy Sources, Part A: Recovery, Utilization, and Environmental Effects*, **43**(9), 1035–1046.
31. Bai, Y., Yang, Z., Zhang, Q., Wei, S., Li, S., & Li, Y. (2020). Preparation of calcium oxide from oyster shell by calcination and its application in biodiesel production. *Energy Conversion and Management*, **207**, 112567.
32. Abdullah, S. H. Y. S., Hanapi, N. H. M., Azid, A., Umar, R., Juahir, H., Khatoon, H., & Endut, A. (2017). A review of biomass-derived heterogeneous catalyst for a sustainable biodiesel production. *Renewable and Sustainable Energy Reviews*, **70**, 1040–1051.
33. Santya, G., Maheswaran, T., & Yee, K. F. (2019). Optimization of biodiesel production from high free fatty acid river catfish oil (Pangasius hypothalamus) and waste cooking oil catalyzed by waste chicken egg shells derived catalyst. *SN Applied Sciences*, **1**(2), 152.
34. Wang, J., Mu, M., & Liu, Y. (2018). Recycled cement. *Construction and Building Materials*, **190**, 1124–1132.
35. Singh, P., Srivastava, S., & Mishra, S. K. (2021). Sustainable calcium oxide production through calcination of limestone: A review. *Journal of Cleaner Production*, **313**, 127965. https://doi.org/10.1016/j.jclepro.2021.127965.
36. Kumar, R., & Yadav, R. (2020). Study of calcination temperature and reaction time of limestone for production of CaO by thermal analysis. *Journal of Thermal Analysis and Calorimetry*, **140**(3), 1463–1474. https://doi.org/10.1007/s10973-019-09125-4.
37. Zhang, Y., Li, X., Zhang, M., Wang, Z., & Liu, G. (2018). Synthesis and characterization of mesoporous calcium oxide from waste shells by calcination. *Journal of Industrial and Engineering Chemistry*, **67**, 193–198. https://doi.org/10.1016/j.jiec.2018.07.024.
38. Jadhav, A., Patil, P., & Bhosale, R. (2020). Doping of calcium oxide for improved catalytic activity: a review. *Journal of Chemical Technology and Biotechnology*, **95**(8), 2077–2089. https://doi.org/10.1002/jctb.6455.
39. Guo, Q., Zhang, Y., Luo, L., & Liu, Y. (2021). Doping of calcium oxide catalysts with copper for efficient biodiesel production from waste cooking oil. *Fuel Processing Technology*, **213**, 106727.
40. Zhang, X., Tang, X., Liu, Y., Zhang, L., & Wang, X. (2020). Co-doping of calcium oxide catalysts with Fe and Zr for biodiesel production. *Fuel Processing Technology*, **204**, 106411. https://doi.org/10.1016/j.fuproc.2020.106411.
41. Naveenkumar, S., & Baskar, G. (2019). Zinc-doped calcium oxide catalyst for transesterification of jatropha oil: Effect of preparation methods. *Journal of Cleaner Production*, **238**, 117867.
42. Cherian, A. J., Remya, N. S., & Jacob, G. (2021). Alumina doped calcium oxide catalyst for biodiesel production from waste cooking oil. *Energy Sources, Part A: Recovery, Utilization, and Environmental Effects*, **43**(9), 1037–1050.
43. Suresh, S., & Toemen, S. (2022). Biodiesel production from waste cooking oil using potassium and chromium doped calcium oxide catalyst. *Journal of Environmental Management*, **303**, 114183.

44. Das, S. K., Nath, S., & Konar, J. (2020). Cobalt-doped calcium oxide catalyst for the transesterification of waste cooking oil: Effect of preparation method. *Energy Sources, Part A: Recovery, Utilization, and Environmental Effects*, **42**(19), 2329–2342.
45. Balakrishnan, P., Kumaravel, A., & T. S. N. (2013). Biodiesel production from jatropha oil using barium doped calcium oxide as heterogeneous catalyst. Journal of Renewable Energy, **53**, 127–134. https://doi.org/10.1016/j.renene.2012.11.027.
46. Martín Alonso, D., Mariscal, R., Rodríguez, F., & Bautista, F. M. (2009). Transesterification of soybean oil over Li-doped CaO catalysts. *Applied Catalysis A: General*, **353**(1), 120–126. https://doi.org/10.1016/j.apcata.2008.11.025.
47. Kesić, Ž., Abazović, N. D., Korać, M., Nikolić, V. B., & Purenović, M. M. (2012). Biodiesel synthesis from sunflower oil over ZnO-doped CaO catalyst prepared by ball milling. *Fuel*, **92**(1), 154–161. https://doi.org/10.1016/j.fuel.2011.08.032.
48. Wu, H., Zhu, S., Xu, Y., & Jiang, Y. (2013). Synthesis of biodiesel over zeolite-supported CaO catalyst under microwave irradiation. *Fuel*, **104**, 702–707. https://doi.org/10.1016/j.fuel.2012.08.027.
49. Moradi, G., Najafpour, G. D., Younesi, H., & Lahijani, P. (2014). Sol-gel synthesis of silicon oxide based calcium oxide nanocatalyst and its application in biodiesel production. *Fuel*, **116**, 665–671. https://doi.org/10.1016/j.fuel.2013.08.066.
50. Arora, R., Nigha, K. S., Verma, P., Wanchoo, R. K., & Toor, A. P. (2024). Microalgal synthesis of the biodiesel employing simultaneous extraction and esterification via heterogeneous catalyst. *Journal of the Indian Chemical Society*, **101**(2), 101123.
51. Kumar, S., Yadav, R., & Sharma, V. (2021). Recent developments in the synthesis of CaO nanomaterials for catalytic applications. *Nano-Structures & Nano-Objects*, **26**, 100669.
52. Liu, Y., Zhang, X., & Yan, S. (2020). Enhancing the catalytic performance of CaO by fabricating a microsphere/nanoparticle composite structure. *Catalysis Science & Technology*, **10**(14), 4672–4682.
53. Ramasamy, M., Ramanathan, M., & Thangamuthu, R. (2021). Influence of surfactant on the morphology and catalytic activity of CaO nanoparticles for transesterification reaction. *Journal of Molecular Liquids*, **333**, 116186.
54. Santos, T. V., Pinto, D. D., Lima, D. F., Tavares, F. W., & Sampaio, J. A. (2022). CaO nanomaterials and their catalytic properties: A review. *Journal of Environmental Chemical Engineering*, **10**(2), 108849.
55. Shu, L., Huang, Y., Zhou, J., Chen, X., & Chen, B. (2021). CaO-based catalysts for CO_2 capture: A review. *Frontiers in Energy Research*, **9**, 702741.
56. Wang, Y., Liu, Y., Zhang, L., Yu, S., & Lu, S. (2020). The effect of morphology on the performance of CaO for CO_2 capture. *Chemical Engineering Journal*, **396**, 125246.
57. Li, J., Liu, X., Zhang, C., & Guo, Y. (2020). Synthesis of alumina-doped CaO nanosheets with improved CO_2 capture performance. *Journal of CO_2 Utilization*, **41**, 101221. https://doi.org/10.1016/j.jcou.2020.101221.
58. Wang, Y., Lu, J., Zhang, Y., Chen, S., Yang, J., & Wu, J. (2021). Zn-doped CaO nanocubes with exposed {001} facets for efficient transesterification of soybean oil. *Applied Surface Science*, **555**, 149523.
59. Kaur, G., Singh, G., & Sharma, P. (2021). Synthesis, characterization and CO_2 capture performance of Ba-doped calcium oxide nanoparticles. Journal of CO_2 Utilization, **48**, 101648. https://doi.org/10.1016/j.jcou.2021.101648.

60. Fu, X., Lin, Q., Zheng, X., & Cai, Y. (2021). Effect of morphology on the catalytic performance of lithium-doped calcium oxide in transesterification of soybean oil. *Catalysts*, **11**(3), 327. https://doi.org/10.3390/catal11030327.
61. Wang, X., Wang, H., Gao, X., & Huang, Q. (2021). Synthesis, characterization, and CO_2 adsorption performance of ZnO-doped CaO nanoparticles. *Journal of Nanoparticle Research*, **23**(3), 87.
62. Sun, C., Zhou, X., Li, Y., Li, B., Huang, Y., Li, J., Li, Q., & Wei, W. (2021). Synthesis and catalytic cracking of heavy oil of CaO-zeolite nanofibers. *Fuel*, **286**, 119530. https://doi.org/10.1016/j.fuel.2020.119530.
63. Kaou, M. H., Horváth, Z. E., Balázsi, K., & Balázsi, C. (2023). Eco-friendly preparation and structural characterization of calcium silicates derived from eggshell and silica gel. *International Journal of Applied Ceramic Technology*, *20*(2), 689–699.
64. Bharti, R., Guldhe, A., Kumar, D., & Singh, B. (2020). Solar irradiation assisted synthesis of biodiesel from waste cooking oil using calcium oxide derived from chicken eggshell. *Fuel*, *273*, 117778.
65. Ferraz, E., Gamelas, J., Coroado, J., Monteiro, C., & Rocha, F. (2020). Exploring the potential of cuttlebone waste to produce building lime. *Materials of Construction*, **70**, e225. https://doi.org/10.3989/mc.2020.15819.
66. Khan, M. D., Ahn, J. W., & Nam, G. (2018). Environmental benign synthesis, characterization and mechanism studies of green calcium hydroxide nano-plates derived from waste oyster shells. *Journal of Environmental Management*, **223**, 947–951.
67. Balaganesh, A.S., Sengodan, R., Ranjithkumar, R., & Chandarshekar, B. (2018). Synthesis and characterization of porous calcium oxide nanoparticles. *International Journal of Innovative Technology and Exploring Engineering (IJITEE)*, **8**(2), 312–314.
68. Kaou, Maroua H., et al. "Eco-friendly preparation and structural characterization of calcium silicates derived from eggshell and silica gel." *International Journal of Applied Ceramic Technology* 20.2 (2023): 689-699.
69. Ferreira, et al. "Chapter 3 - Waste Biorefinery." Sustainable Resource Recovery and Zero Waste Approaches 2019, Pages 35–52.
70. Rupam Bharti, Abhishek Guldhe, Dipesh Kumar, Bhaskar Singh "Solar irradiation assisted synthesis of biodiesel from waste cooking oil using calcium oxide derived from chicken eggshell" *Fuel*, Volume 273, 1 August 2020, 117778.

Index